*Martial Art
History, Forms and T*
Volume Two

Kang Duk Won

The Korean Contribution

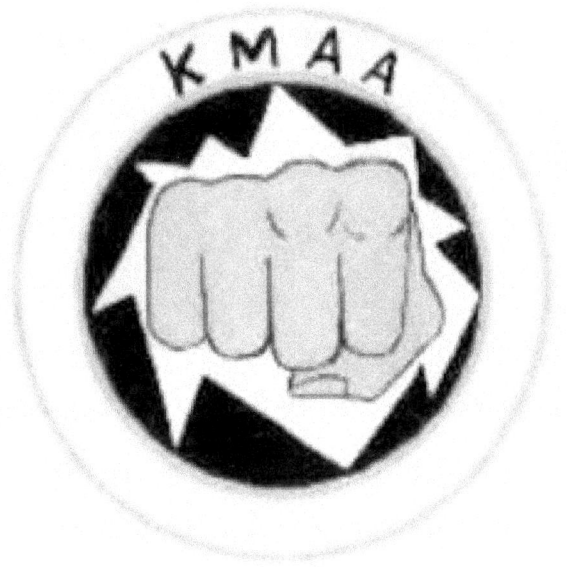

by
Al Case

AL CASE

Quality Press

Copyright© 2024 Alton H. Case
All rights reserved.

All rights reserved. No part of this book may be reproduced or transmitted in any form or by any means, electronic or mechanical, including photocopying, recording, or by any information storage and retrieval system, without the written permission of the author.

For information regarding this book go to:

MonsterMartialArts.com
or
AlCaseBooks.com

KANG DUK WON

TABLE OF CONTENTS

	introduction	5
1	pinan one	7
2	pinan two	22
3	pinan three	43
4	pinan four	57
5	pinan five	81
6	sip su	105
7	no hai	128
8	bot sai	147
9	um be	172
10	kima shodan	189
	about the author	194

AL CASE

INTRODUCTION

Kang Duk Won translates as 'House for Espousing Virtue.'

It was originally a form of Korean Karate taught by a fellow name of Byung In Joon. It was the choice of three Imperial Guards for three different countries.

It was influenced by Tong Bei Chinese internal gung fu.

It is a 'pre-Funakoshi' art, which makes it one of the purest forms of Karate in the world.

Here is a brief description leading to the Kang Duk Won.

Byung In Joon was a Korean lad who wanted to learn martial arts.

He found a Chinese martial arts instructor, and begged for instruction. He was turned down.

Not to be stopped, Byung would line up the shoes of the students on the front step while they were in class. The old Chinese master was curious about who would do such a thing, and, when he found out who it was, he accepted Bung as a student.

Byung spent many years learning his martial arts, but eventually he was sent away for advanced education.

At the university, he would practice his martial arts by hitting a tree, which tree began to slant over.

One day a Korean classmate ran up to him followed by several Japanese.

"I joined their Karate class, but now I have a girlfriend and don't want to go! You know martial arts! You've got to protect me!"

Byung faced the Japanese karate students and told them there would be no fight.

The students came at him, and he managed to fend them off without hurting any of them.

The master who taught these Japanese Karate students was quite curious concerning this fellow who could defeat his students without harming them, and went to meet him. His name was Kanken Toyama.

Byung and the old Karate master decided to trade systems. In a short while Byung was teaching the class, and he was awarded high rank and teaching credentials.

Byung returned home and began teaching Karate. He was instrumental in the development of the five Kwans that made up the original Korean Karate associations. These kwans later became the foundation for Taekwondo.

Unfortunately for Byung, the Korean war began. His brother was a captain in the North Korean army, and he commanded Byung to come to the north with him.

Byung fought through the war, and was eventually imprisoned. When Koreans were allowed by the Americans to return to their homes, the North Koreans would not allow Byung to leave.

Byung spent the remainder of his life working in a cement factory, where he apparently contracted a lung disease. Poor, physically broken, one of the greatest masters of Karate returned home to die.

In the meantime, the people he had taught had developed their kwans, and Korean Karate began to spread. From Byung in Joon the art was transmitted to Park Chulhee, and then to Norman Rha, and finally to Bob Babich.
Sensei Babich taught the Kang Duk Won in San Jose, and brought the art to its highest form.

Sensei Babich taught Al Case, who wrote this book.

The Kang Duk Won is a pure form of Karate, what is called a 'closed combat system.'
This book presents the system as Al Case originally learned it, with no changes to the forms he learned back in the late 60s and early 70s.

If you are a serious student of Karate, and you wish to see the potential differences between the Karate you study, and Karate the way it was taught back in the sixties, when it first came out of Korea and into the United States, then this is the book for you.
It includes the ten basic forms of the Kang Duk Won, and the fifty original techniques.

PINAN ONE

The Pinan forms are considered the base of Okinawan/Japanese (classical) Karate. Pinan means 'Peaceful Mind.' One who knows the Pinans can be considered to have a peaceful mind. Also, one who knows the Pinans can be considered to have graduated from 'high school' in Karate. Here is the first form...Pinan One.

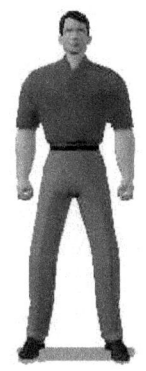 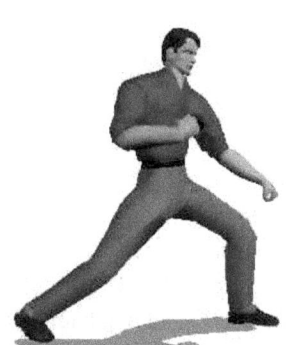

Stand in a natural stance stance. The fists should be loosely closed. The attitude and balance should be that of a person who can move instantly in any direction.

Step to the left with the left foot into a front stance, simultaneously execute a left low block.

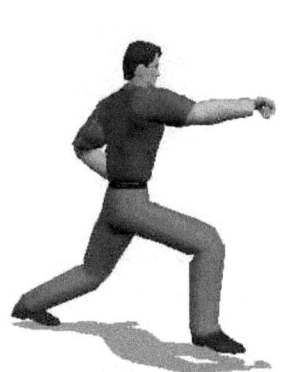 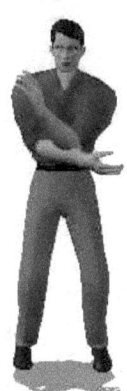

Step forward with the right foot into a front stance, simultaneously execute a right punch.

Step back with the right foot. This is a transitional move through the original position. Note the position of the hands for blocking.

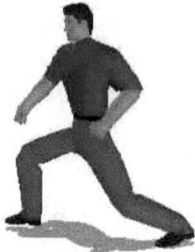 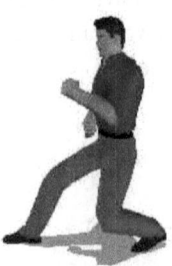

Step to the right with the right foot, simultaneously execute a right low block.

Step back with the right foot into a back stance, simultaneously begin rolling the left hand in a hammerfist. While it is transitional, the hammerfist should be very real.

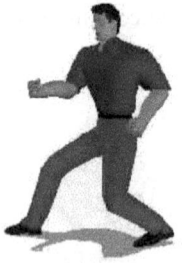 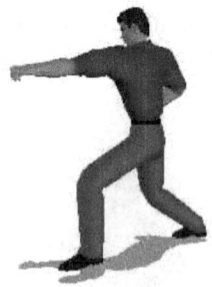

Continue rolling the hands so as to execute a right hammerfist. The forearm should be level with the floor, and the hips should be turned to the right so that the body aligns.

Step forward with the left foot into a front stance, simultaneously execute a left punch.

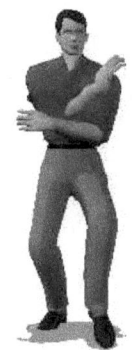 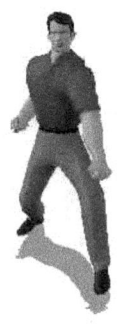

Retract the left foot and face to the left in a cat stance. Guard the face with the right palm and prepare the left palm.

Step forward with the left foot into a front stance, simultaneously execute a left low block. Examine how the shoulders turn (and hips) so that the body achieves perfect alignment.

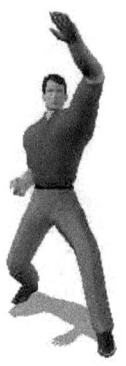 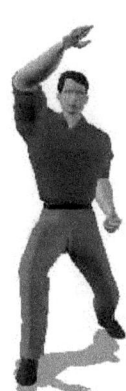

Retract the left foot and assume a back stance as you execute a left high knife block.

Step forward with the right foot into a front stance while simultaneously executing a right high block.

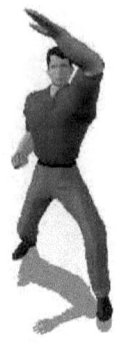 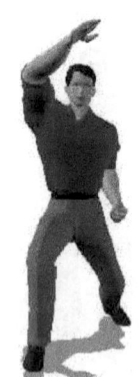

Step forward with the left foot into a front stance while simultaneously executing a left high block.

Step forward with the right foot into a front stance while simultaneously executing a right punch.

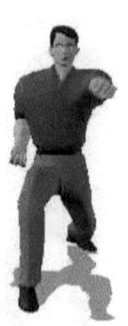 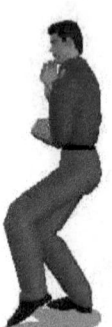

Execute a punch with the left hand. KIAI!

Retract the left foot and pivot 90 degress to the rear. (The left foot will go behind you.) Simultaneously prepare the hands. This is a transitional move.

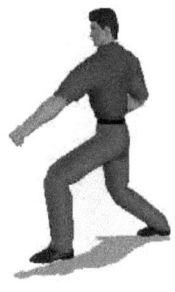 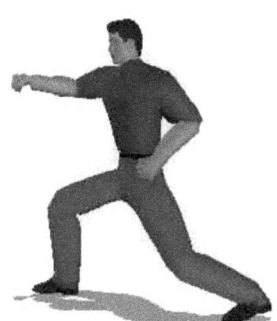

Step forward with the left foot into a front stance, simultaneously execute a left low block.

Step forward with the right foot into a front stance, simultaneously executing a right punch.

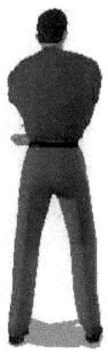 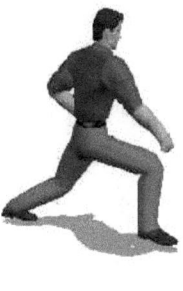

Step back with the right foot. This is a transitional move through the original position, don't stop and pose but move through without grounding. Note the position of the hands for blocking. (This is exactly the same position as the fourth picture in this form)

Continue stepping to the right with the right foot as you execute a right low block.

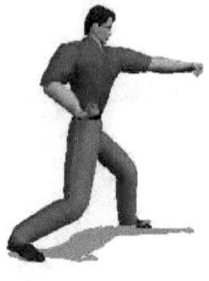 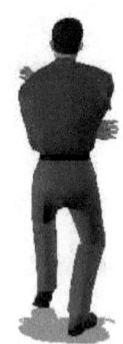

Step forward with the left foot as you execute a left front punch.

Retract the left foot and face to the left in a cat stance. Guard the face with the right palm and prepare the left palm. (This is exactly the same as picture eight in this form.)

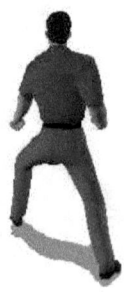 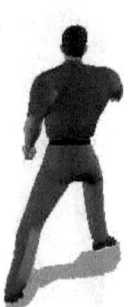

Step forward with the left foot into a front stance as you execute a left low block.

Step forward with the right foot as you execute a right punch.

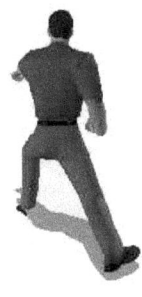 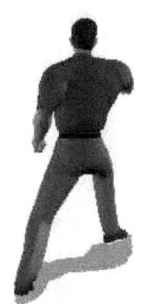

Step forward with the right foot as you execute a left punch.
Step forward with the left foot as you execute a right punch. KIAI!

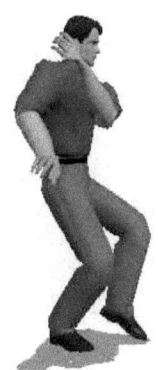 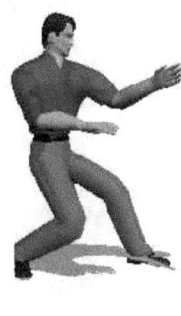

Swing the left foot 90 degrees behind you as you pivot to face to the right. Assume a cat stance with the arms prepared for a double knife block. This is a transitional move.

Move the left foot forward and assume a back stance as you execute a left double knife block.

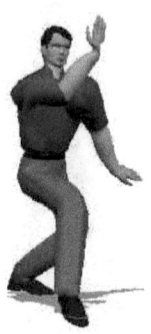 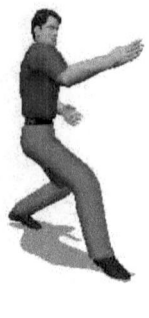

  Move the right foot forward and to the right through a transitional cat stance as you prepare the arms for a right double knife block.
  Assume a right back stance as you execute a right double knife block. (The difference between a double knife and a single knife is that in a double knife both hands move into the block, in the single knife the back hand moves away from the block.)

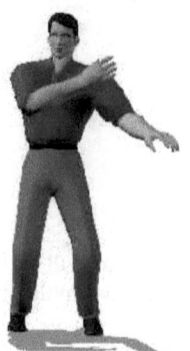 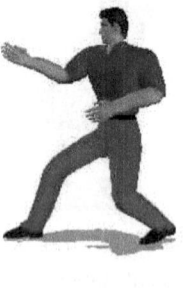

  Move the right foot back to a transitional natural stance with the arms prepared for a double knife.
  Finish pivoting to the right into a back stance as you execute a right double knife block.

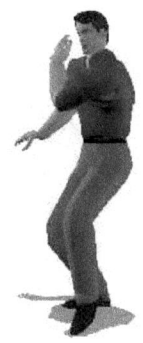 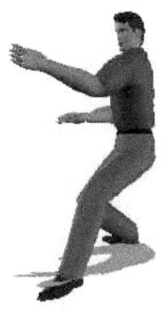

Move the left foot forward and to the left through a transitional cat stance as you prepare the arms for a left double knife block.

Move the left foot forward into a back stance as you execute a left double knife block.

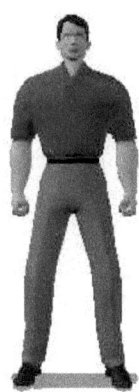

Retract the left foot to a natural stance. You should be at the position where you began the form.

A simple form, yes? Definitely Karate. not to be confused with Kung Fu. Not even closely resembling Aikido. Yet...if you are going to Matrix your art, you should understand one simple fact, All Arts are the Same!

APPLICATION NUMBER ONE

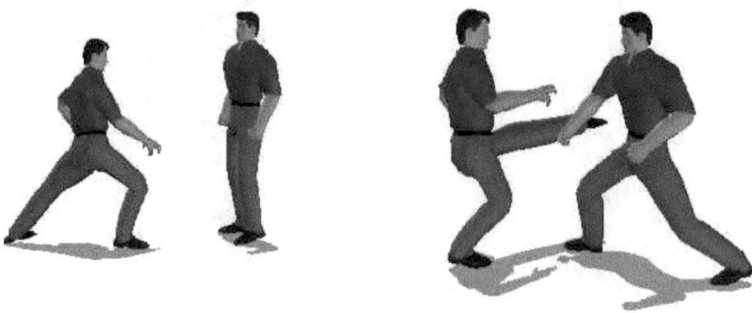

The Attacker prepares to kick.

The Attacker launches a left kick to the groin. The Defender steps back with the left foot into a front stance as he executes a right low block.

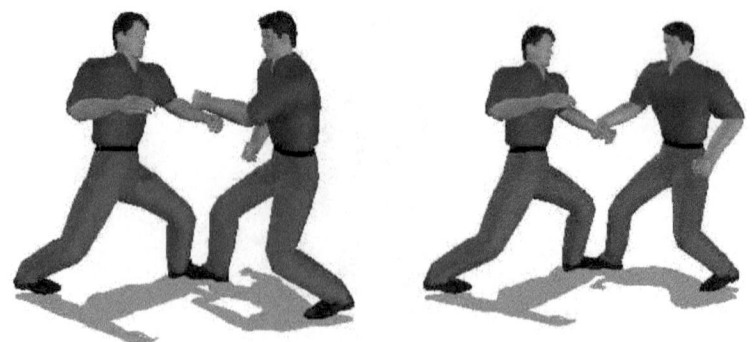

The Attacker sets his left foot down in a front stance as he executes a left punch to the body. The Defender shifts back into a back stance as he rolls a right hammerfist on the Attacker's left fist.

The Defender rolls his hands to strike the Attacker's left fist with his right fist. While this doesn't appear very realistic, with practice it is possible to punch somebody's fist in the middle of their attack. It does take practice, and this technique will increase hand speed tremendously. Don't forget to shift the hips slightly on the hand roll so that the body is always aligned.

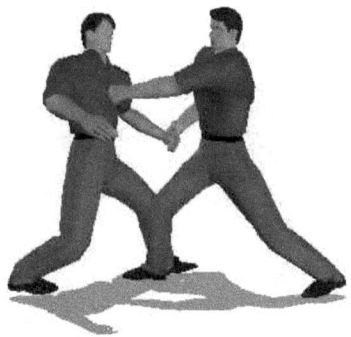

The Defender shifts forward (stepping, if necessary, with the right foot) as he executes a left punch to the chest.

The three elements of power are thrusting the weight forward, rotating the hips, and dropping the weight. Can you figure out how much of each element of power is put into each movement of the defense?

APPLICATION NUMBER TWO

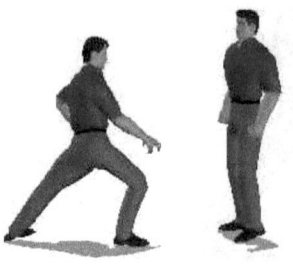 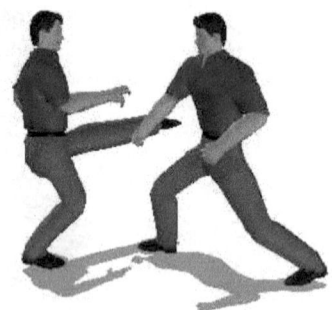

The Attacker prepares to kick.
The Attacker launches a left kick to the groin. The Defender steps back with the left foot into a front stance as he executes a right low block.

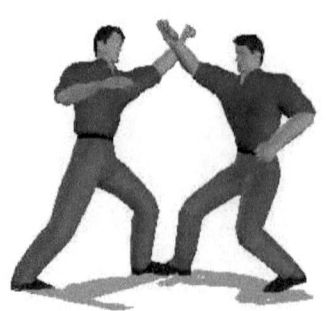 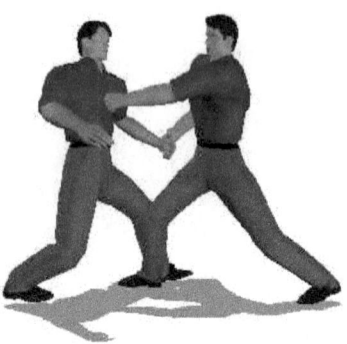

The Attacker sets his left foot down in a front stance as he executes a left punch to the face. The Defender shifts back into a back stance as he executes a right high knife hand. Remember to bring the elbow of the knife hand in and to drive the knife hand like an uppercut up the centerline of the body. This will better enable you to snap the elbow out and into the block.

The Defender shifts forward (stepping, if necessary, with the right foot) as he executes a left punch to the chest.
The three elements of power are thrusting the weight forward, rotating the hips, and dropping the weight. Can you figure out how much of each element of power is put into each movement of the defense?

APPLICATION NUMBER THREE

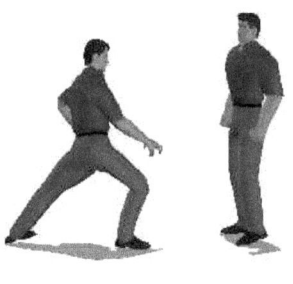 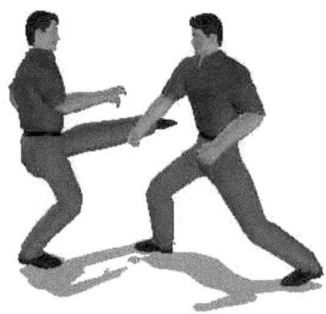

The Attacker prepares to kick.

The Attacker launches a left kick to the groin. The Defender steps back with the left foot into a front stance as he executes a right low block.

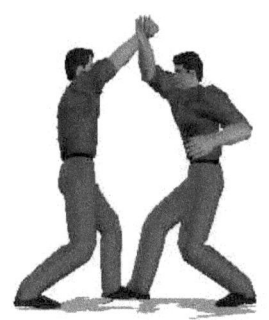 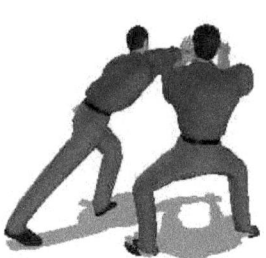

The Attacker sets his left foot down in a front stance as he executes a left punch to the face. The Defender shifts back into a back stance as he executes a right high knife hand. Remember to bring the elbow of the knife hand in and to drive the knife hand like an uppercut up the centerline of the body. This will better enable you to snap the elbow out and into the block.

The Defender steps forward as he places the right hand on the defender's elbow and executes an armbar.

You can take this application to a lot of different places now. You can step into his armpit and start elbowing his head or ribs, and maybe spike his back (an old Kenpo technique), or you can whirl him around (spinning him like an airplane, as in Aikido) or you can drop him down, step over his arm and fall back (as in Ju Jitsu). The purpose of these applications is not to tell you the only way you can do something, but to open the door so that you can do anything.

APPLICATION NUMBER FOUR

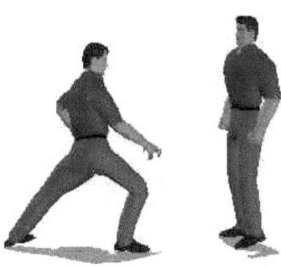 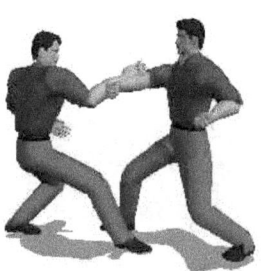

The Attacker prepares to punch.

The Attacker steps forward with the left foot into a front stance as he punches to the chest with the left hand. The Defender steps back with the left foot into a back stance as he executes a right double knife block.

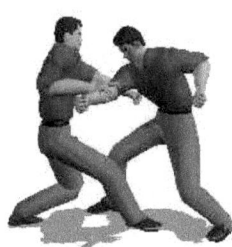

The Defender grabs the Attacker's left wrist with his right hand and pulls back slightly as he executes a left punch to the axilla. (Look up axilla in a dictionary.)

The pull is slight, but done with the full body weight. The idea is not to pull the attacker over, but to introduce enough body weight so he can't drop an elbow to block, and thus the axilla is revealed. (I told you to look that word up in a dictionary!)

PINAN TWO

An interesting tidbit about Pinan Two is that it was originally taught before Pinan One. Eventually someone realized that two was easier than one, and so switched the order so that they would be taught in proper sequence. Before we start this form, check out the picture below, it is a picture of Mr. Funakoshi leading a class in a form called 'Pinan Shodan.' Looks like Pinan Two, to me.

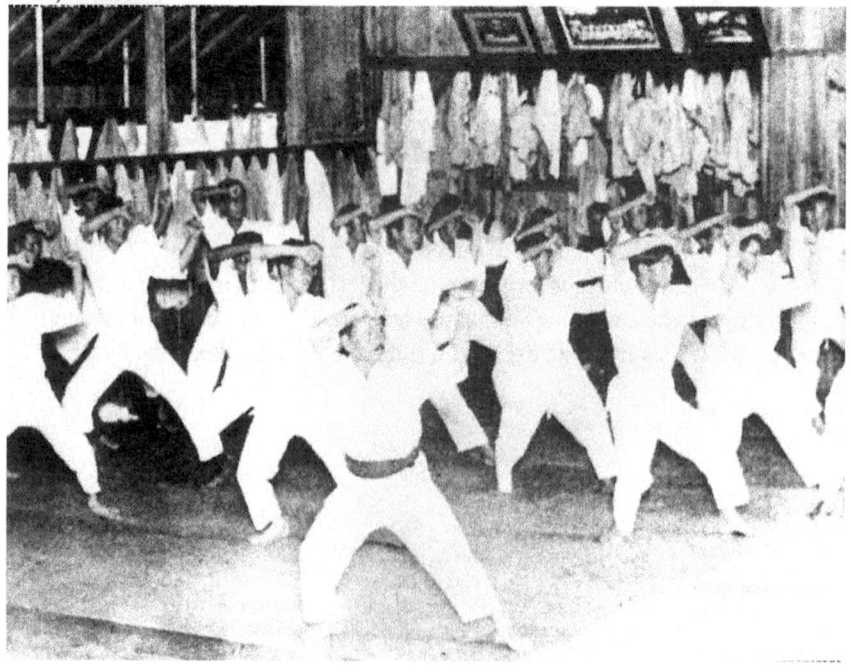

The first move of Pinan Two is on the following page.

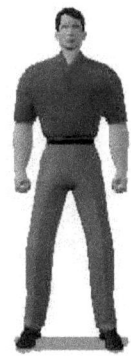 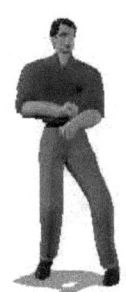

Stand in a natural stance stance. The fists should be loosely closed. The attitude and balance should be that of a person who can move instantly in any direction.

Start to pivot to the left and raise the hands so that the back of the right fist back is over the back of the left fist. (Putting the fists back to back will set up wrist snapping at the end of this move. This is an important point to remember in nearly all of the moves of the forms)

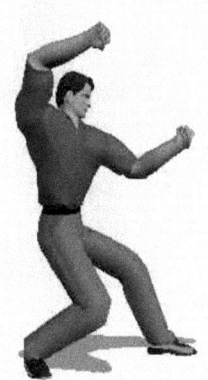 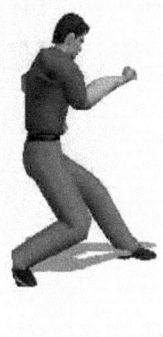

Extend the left foot into a back stance as you execute a left outward middle block and a right high block.

Retract the left hand to the hip as you execute a right inward middle block.

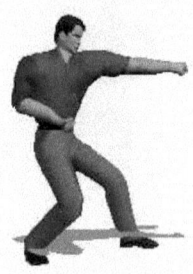 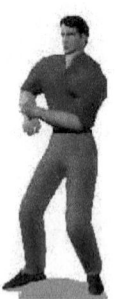

Retract the right hand to the hip as you execute a left punch.

Start pivoting to the right and raise the hands so that the back of the left fist is over the back of the right fist.

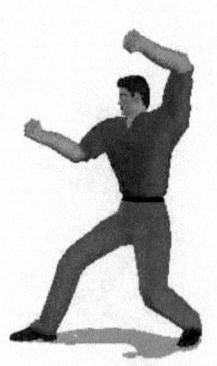 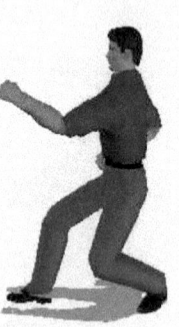

Extend the left foot into a back stance as you execute a right outward middle block and a left high block.

Retract the right arm to the hip as you execute a left inward middle block.

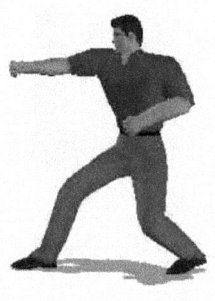 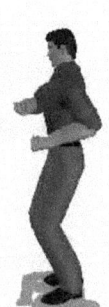

Retract the left arm to the hip as you execute a right punch. Make sure you pivot the hips slightly so that the body is fully aligned in each move.

Move the left foot forward and place it next to the right foot. The right arm bends so that the upper arm is at forty-five degrees and the elbow is at ninety degrees.

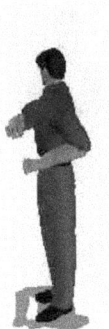 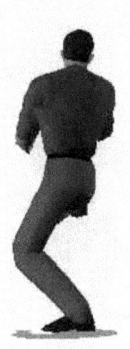

Stand up slowly, turning your face to the right as you do so.

The feet should be exactly side by side (I didn't quite make this happen in this picture.) This is called 'marrying the feet.'

Execute a simultaneous right snap kick and a right outward middle block. Make sure you lock the block and snap the kick.

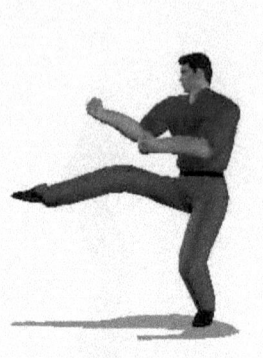 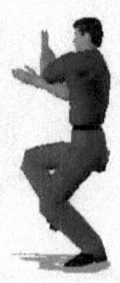

side view of above.

The next move is tricky. You must pivot to the left, stomp the right foot and execute a left double knife block. This all must be done simultaneously. One thing that will help is to keep the hips centered. I am showing this in two moves, the transition (let the hands circle over) and the final double knife block. The sudden stomping of the foot increases the weight, which requires more work, or power. Thus, the technique is 'supercharged.'

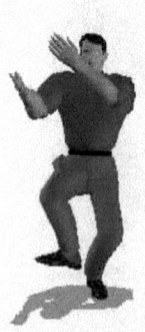 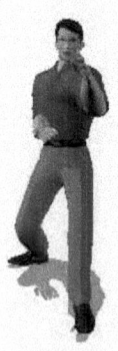

Side view of above.

The final position is a back stance with a double knife block. Make sure you utilize gravity throughout your whole body to power this move.

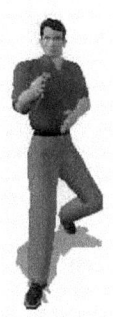 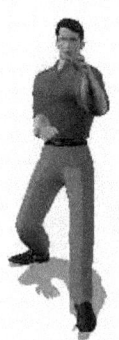

Step forward with the right foot into a back stance as you execute a right double knife block. Make sure you bring the hands over and down with just the right amount of diagonal direction.

Step forward with the left foot into a back stance as you execute a left double knife block.

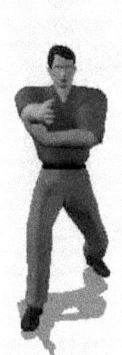 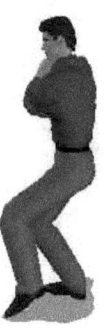

Step forward with the right foot into a front stance as you execute a right spearhand and a left cross palm block. KIAI!

This next sequence of four moves is the same as that of the last four moves in Pinan One. Bring the left foot behind the right foot and travel through a transitional cat while preparing the hands for a double knife. The angle is 90 degrees to the rear. While this is shorter than 270 around the front, it seems a bit blind to be moving in this fashion. Can you think of a better way to set up this sequence of four moves?

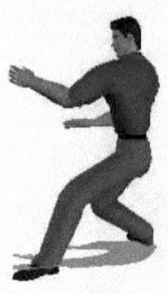 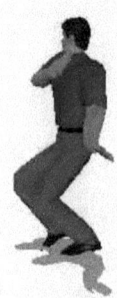

Extend the left foot into a back stance as you execute a left double knife block.

Step forward and to the right with the right foot. This is a transitional cat stance, and the arms should be preparing for a right double knife.

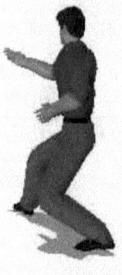 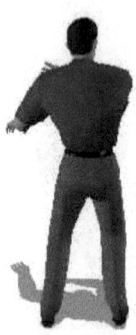

Assume a right back stance as you execute a right double knife block.

Step back with the right foot to the previous position and prepare the arms for a right double knife block.

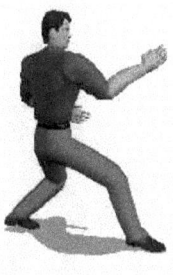 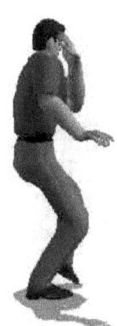

Assume a right back stance as you execute a right double knife block.
Step forward and to the left with the left foot. This is a transitional cat stance, and the arms should be preparing for a left double knife.

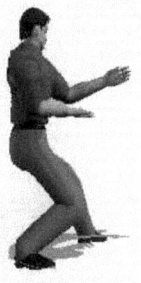 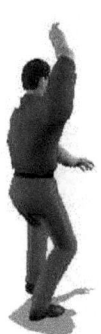

Assume a left back stance as you execute a left double knife block.
Bring the left foot back to a cat as you execute a left low block and a right high block. This is a transitional stance and the movements should not be focused, but just the start of circling the arms.

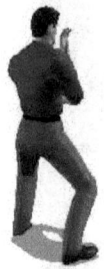 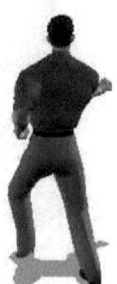

Step with the left foot to the left (ninety degrees) as you continue circling the arms through a 'Buddha Palm' block. The left hand is in a palm and the right hand is scooping under the elbow.

Plant the weight on the left foot as you turn the hips into a right outward block. This block can be a block, or an uppercut.

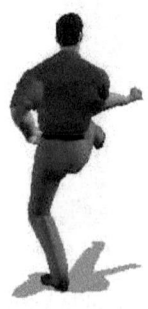 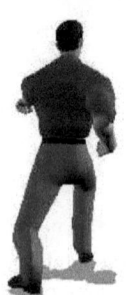

Right front snap kick
Set the right foot forward in a front stance as you execute a left punch.

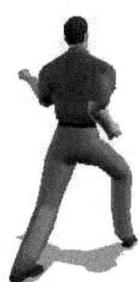 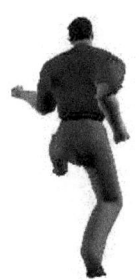

Move the left foot slightly forward as you twist the hips (and the left foot, so it points towards the right foot) and execute a left outward middle block. Left front snap kick.

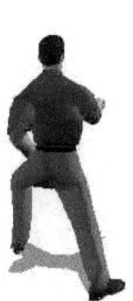 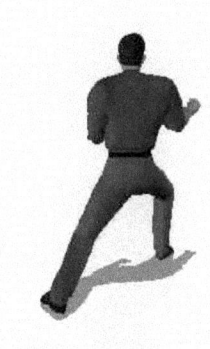

Set the right foot down in a front stance as you execute a left punch.
Step forward with the right foot into a front stance as you execute a right outward middle block. KIAI!

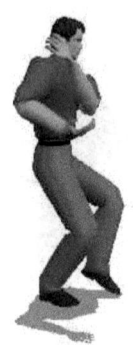 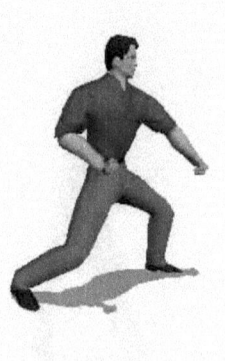

Move the left foot behind the right foot (ninety degrees) into a cat stance as you prepare the arms for a low block. Do not focus as this is a transitional move.

Step forward with the left foot into a front stance as you execute a left low block.

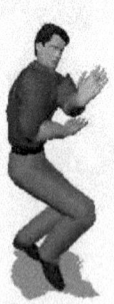 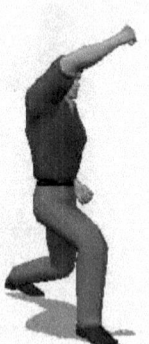

Step forward and to the right with the right foot into a cat stance as you prepare for a high block. the arms should be in a 'Buddha Palm' position, with the left hand cross paling and the right hand scooping under the elbow.

Step forward with the right foot into a front stance as you execute a right high block. Remember to move the right arm up the centerline of the body and then snap the elbow outwards.

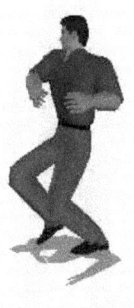 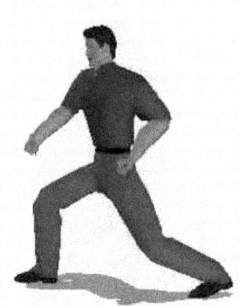

Step back to the previous position as you pivot 135 degrees to the right. Assume a cat stance as you retract the right arm for a low block. This is a transitional stance.

Step forward with the left foot into a front stance as you execute a left low block.

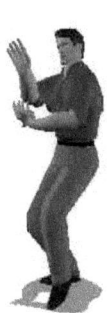 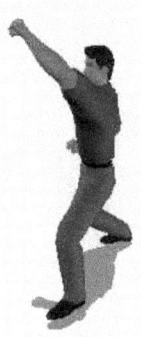

Step forward and to the left with the right foot into a cat stance as you prepare for a right high block. The cat stance should be transitional, and the hands should travel through the 'Buddha Palm' position.

Step forward with the left foot into a front stance as you execute a left high block.

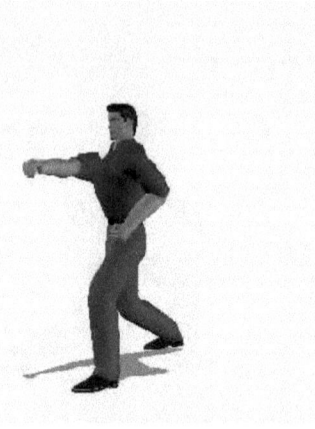 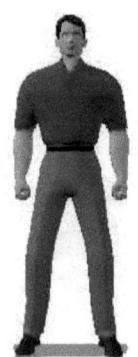

Execute a right punch. KIAI!

Step back with the left foot to a natural stance (to the beginning position of the form).

APPLICATION NUMBER FIVE

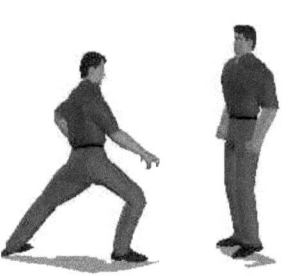 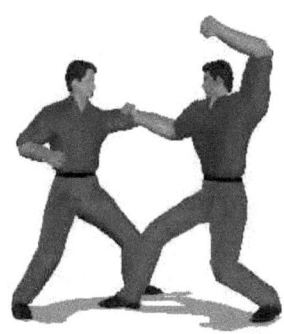

The Attacker prepares to punch.
The Attacker steps forward with the left foot into a front stance as he punches to the chest with the left hand. The Defender steps back with the right foot into a front stance as he executes a right outward middle block and a left high block.

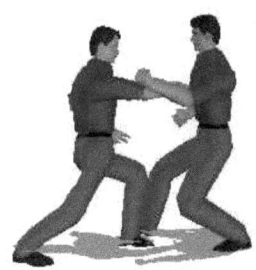 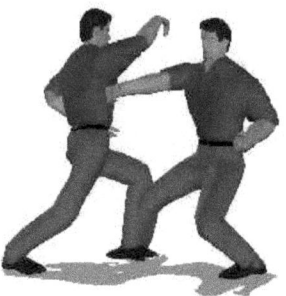

The Attacker punches to the chest with the right hand. The Defender pivots to the right as he executes a left inward middle block.
The Defender pivots to the left as he executes a punch to the chest.
I call this the 'Hidden Fist' technique. When you punch your fist should go under the arm of the attacker, thus being hidden from his view.

While you can strike anywhere on the barrel, it is best to strike right in the axilla. Make sure you look up axilla in the dictionary.

APPLICATION NUMBER SIX

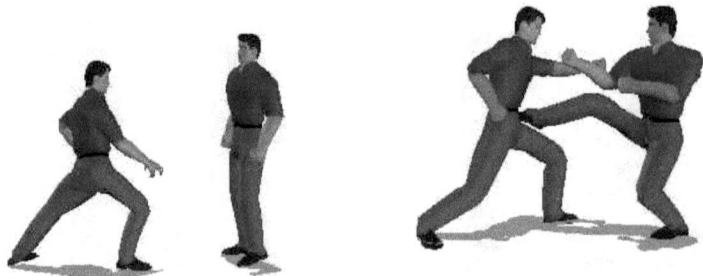

The Attacker prepares to punch.

The Attacker steps forward with the left foot into a front stance as he punches to the chest with the left hand. The Defender executes a right snap kick to the stomach and a right outward middle block.

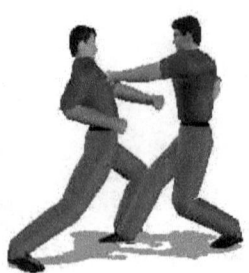

The Defender sets his right foot down in a back stance as he executes a left punch. (If distance must be closed the Defender should shuffle.)

I call this technique 'Stop Kick.' This is because the kick should be fast enough to stop the attacker.

I like giving names to the techniques, whenever possible, because it makes them easier to remember

APPLICATION NUMBER SEVEN

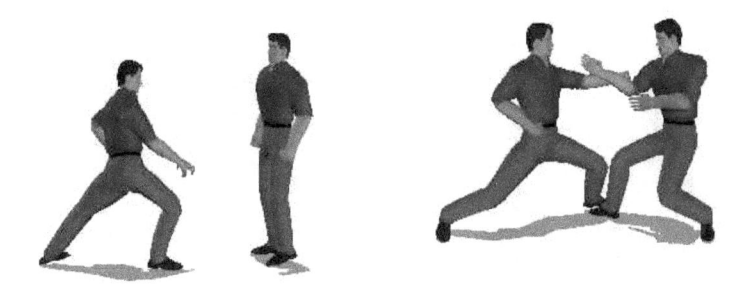

The Attacker prepares to punch.

The Attacker steps forward with the left foot into a front stance as he punches to the chest with the left hand. The Defender steps back with the right foot as he executes a left double knife block.

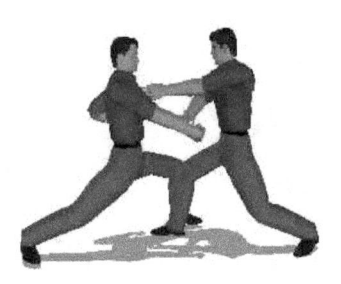

The Attacker punches with the right hand. The Defender shifts forward into a front stance as he executes a right cross palm block (or 'smother' block) and a left spear hand to the solar plexus.

APPLICATION NUMBER EIGHT

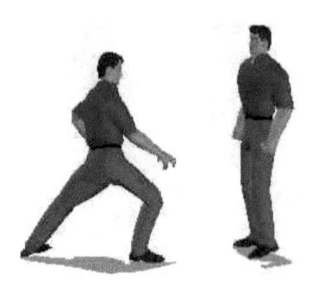

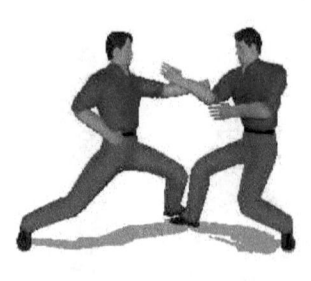

The Attacker prepares to punch.

The Attacker steps forward with the left foot into a front stance as he punches to the chest with the left hand. The Defender steps back with the right foot as he executes a left double knife block.

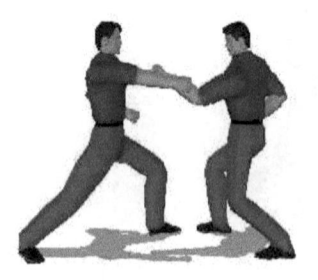

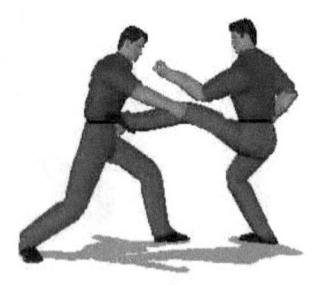

The Attacker punches with the right hand. The Defender twists to the right as he executes a left outward middle block. The front leg should be placed (usually drawn back) so that there is enough room for the next move, a kick to the solar plexus.

The Defender executes a left snap kick to the solar plexus.

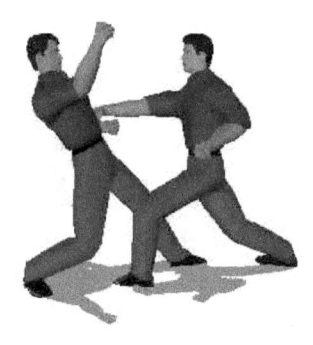

The Defender sets the left foot forward in a front stance as he executes a left punch.

I call this 'Twist and Kick.'

APPLICATION NUMBER TEN

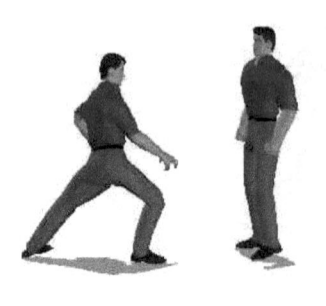

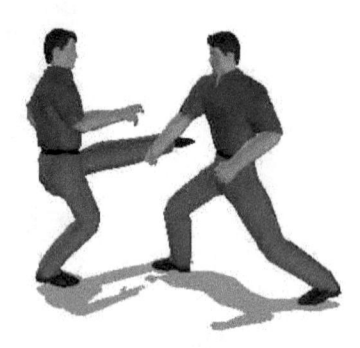

The Attacker prepares to kick.
The Attacker executes a left front snap kick. The Defender steps back with the left foot into a front stance (thereby dropping his weight into the block) as he executes a right low block.

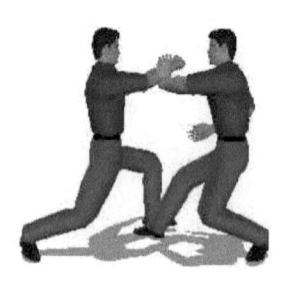

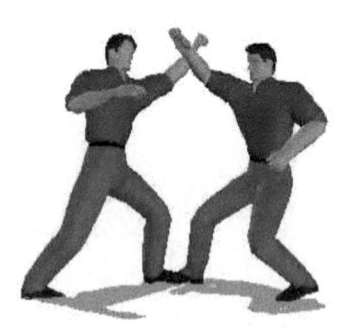

The Attacker executes a left punch to the face. The Defender shifts back to a back stance as he executes a left cross palm block.
The Attacker executes a left punch to the face. The Defender executes a right high block. (Remember to shift the hips so that the body is aligned on each movement of this application.)

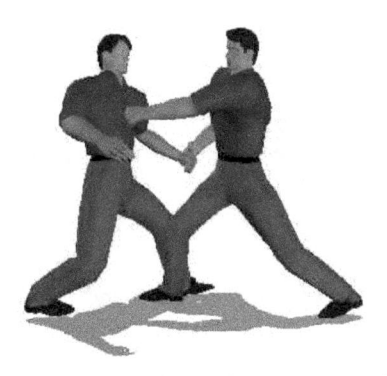

The Defender shifts forward into a front stance as he executes a left punch to the body.

APPLICATION NUMBER NINE

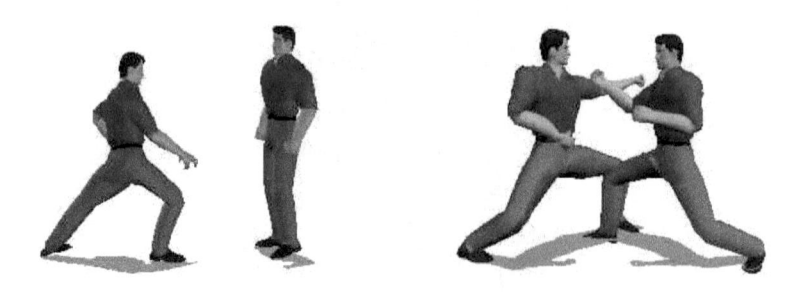

The Attacker prepares to punch.

The Attacker steps forward with the left foot into a front stance as he punches to the chest with the left hand. The Defender steps forward with the right foot as he executes a right outward middle block. The Defender must learn how to move first and fastest. This is done by practicing the applications until one develops a certain intuition in these matters.

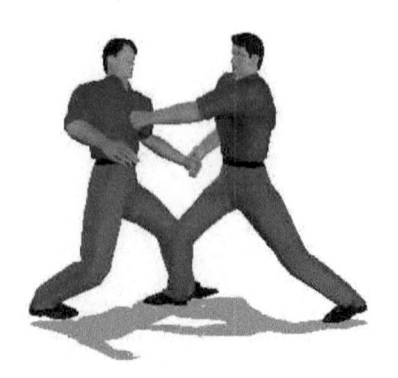

The Defender executes a left punch. The power comes from a slight twist of the hips.

PINAN THREE

Pinan three is a shorter form than the other Pinans, but it introduces the horse stance and some good throws.

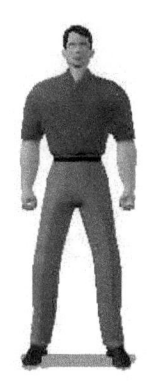

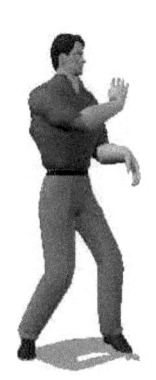

Stand in a natural stance stance. The fists should be loosely closed. The attitude and balance should be that of a person who can move instantly in any direction.

Start pivoting to the left. The left hand should stay where it is and 'dangle' in a parry, and the right hand should slide through a cross palm block to cover the face. This is a transitional move.

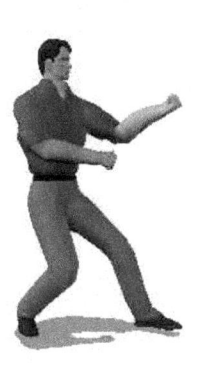

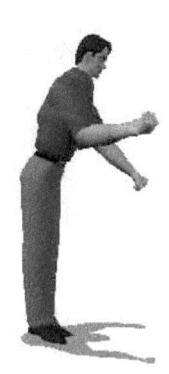

Complete the pivot to the left into a back stance as you execute a left outward middle block. There should be a subtle shifting of the hips to create internal power.

Place the right foot next to the left, straighten the knees and lean forward as you execute a right outward middle block and a left low block.

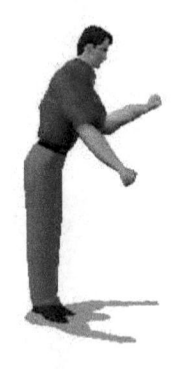

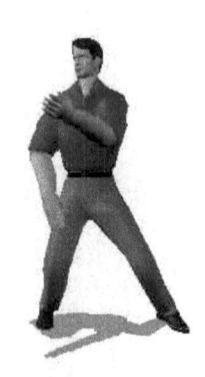

Bring the hands back slightly and pass them through a back of the fist to a back of the fist position on the way to a left outward middle block and a right low block. The reason this is important because most moves in a karate form should set up a 'fist twist' to increase focus and power.

Move the left foot backwards and start pivoting to the right. The right hand should move to a 'dangle' parry, and the left hand should slide through a cross palm block to cover the face. This is a transitional move.

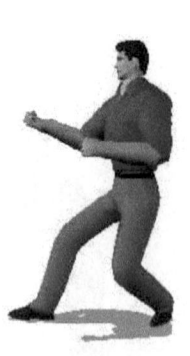

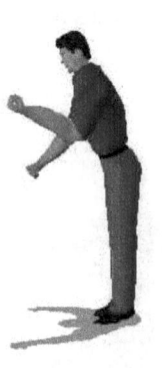

Complete the pivot to the right into a back stance as you execute a right outward middle block. There should be a subtle shifting of the hips to create internal power.

Place the left foot next to the right, straighten the knees and lean forward as you execute a left outward middle block and a right low block.

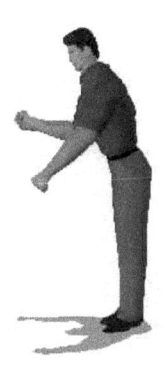

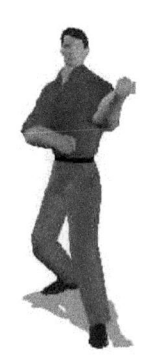

Bring the hands back slightly and pass them through a back of the fist to a back of the fist position on the way to a right outward middle block and a left low block.

Step to the left with the left foot into a back stance as you execute a left outward middle block.

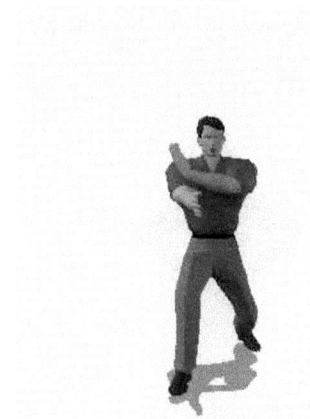

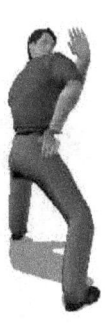

Step forward with the right foot into a front stance as you execute a right spear hand and a left cross palm block to cover the face.

Pivot to the rear and step to the left with the left foot so that you are in a front stance facing in the opposite direction. Lean slightly as you retract the right hand to a parry position against the kidney and cover the face with a left cross palm block.

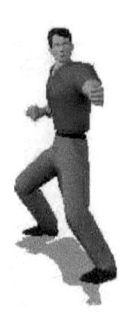

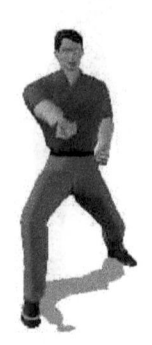

Step back towards the front of the form with the left foot (thus completing a circle with the footwork) into a horse stance as you execute a left backfist. The right hand should be in a loose fist, cocked at the hip. All fists should always be loose, except for as brief a moment as possible when focusing on a strike or block.

Step forward with the right foot into a front stance as you execute a right punch.

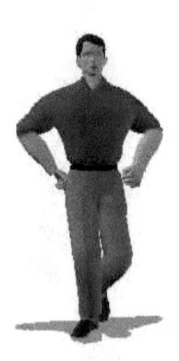

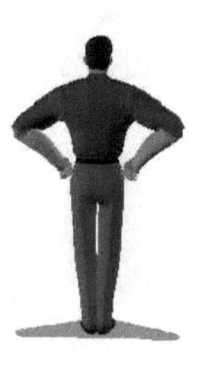

Place the toe of the left foot behind the heel of the right.

Pivot to the rear as you place the fists on the hips with the elbows to the side. This pivot should be done without unduly moving the feet.

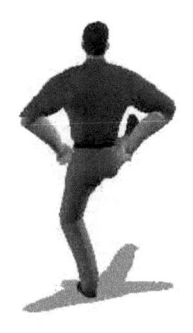

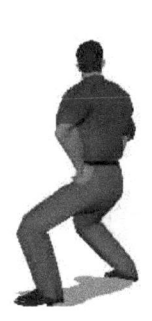

Execute a right leg raise. Make sure you keep the hips low on this movement.

Set the right foot down in a horse stance as you execute a block with the right elbow.

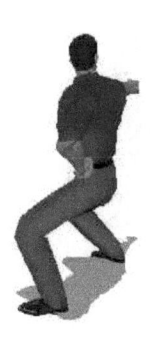

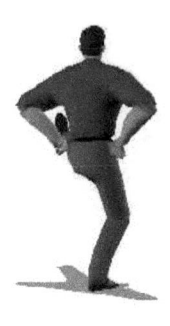

Execute a right backfist. Make sure you snap the backfist hard and fast and return it to the fist on the hips position.

Execute a left leg raise. Again, very important to keep the hips low on this movement.

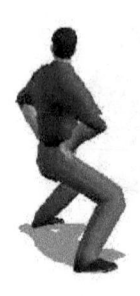

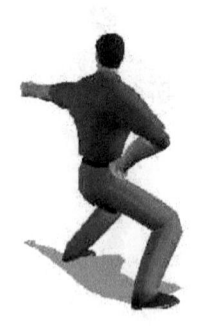

Set the left foot down in a horse stance as you execute a block with the left elbow.

Execute a left backfist. Again, snap it hard and return it to the fist on the hips position.

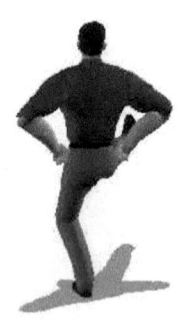

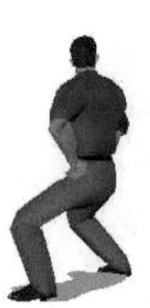

Execute a right leg raise. Keep those durned hips low.

Set the right leg down in a horse stance as you execute a right elbow block.

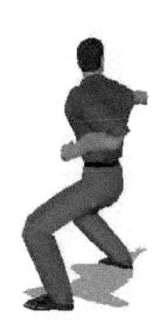

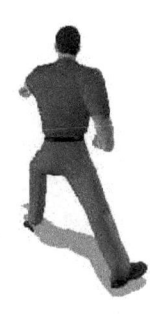

Execute a right backfist. This time lock it, and retract the left elbow to a cocked position at the hip.

Step forward with the left foot to a front stance as you execute a left punch.

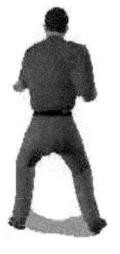

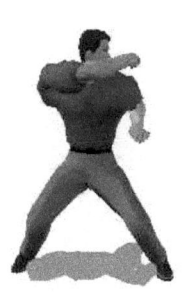

Bring the right foot forward until it is next to the left foot but shoulder distance apart.

Step behind the right foot with the left foot and spin into a horse stance as you execute a right fist over the shoulder and a left elbow spike to the rear.

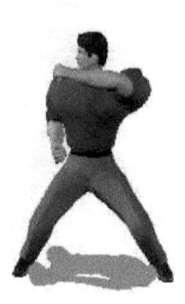

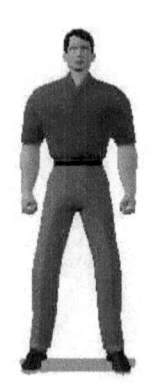

Shuffle to the right into a horse stance as you execute a left fist over the shoulder and right elbow spike to the rear.

Retract the right foot to the left and return to the natural position.

APPLICATION NUMBER ELEVEN

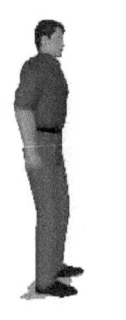

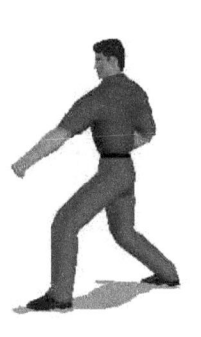

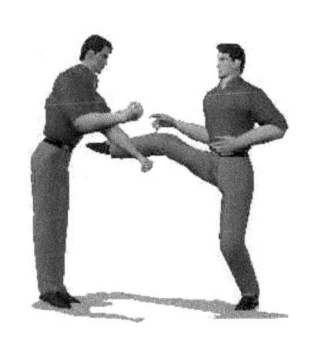

The Attacker prepares to kick.
The Attacker executes a right snap kick to the belly.

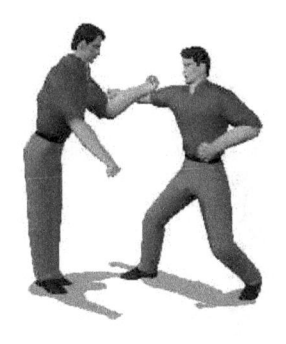

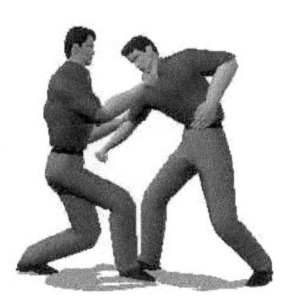

    The Attacker steps forward with the right foot into a front stance as he punches to the chest with the right hand. The Defender executes a left outward middle block and a right low block.

    The Defender places the right foot next to the left foot as he pulls the Attacker's right hand with his left hand and executes a right uppercut to the throat.

    The lesson behind this technique is that you can rearrange the movements of the form to make other applications.

APPLICATION NUMBER TWELVE

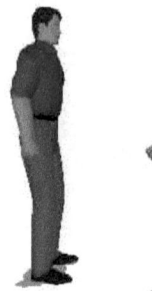

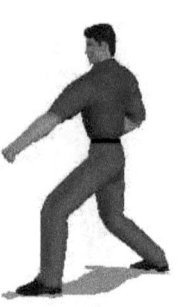

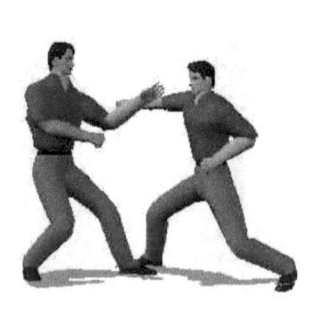

The Attacker prepares to punch.

The Attacker steps forward with the right foot into a front stance as he punches to the chest with the right hand. The Defender steps back with the right foot as he executes a left outward middle block.

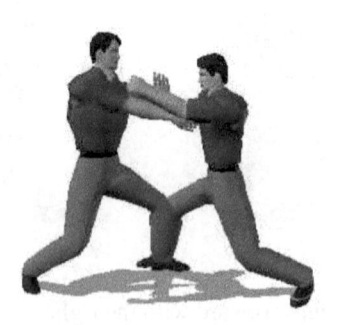

The Attacker executes a left punch to the face. The Defender shifts forward into a front stance as he executes a left cross palm block and a right spearhand to the solar plexus.

The difference between this one and the application out of Pinan Two is that the Defender must move forward into a punch directed at his face. This calls for more confront and better timing.

I call this one Spear Under.

APPLICATION NUMBER THIRTEEN

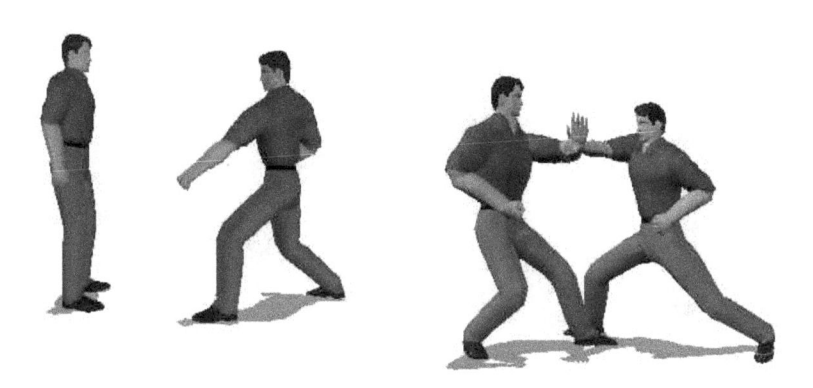

The Attacker prepares to punch.

The Attacker steps forward with the right foot into a front stance as he punches to the chest with the right hand. The Defender steps back with the right foot as he executes a left cross palm block.

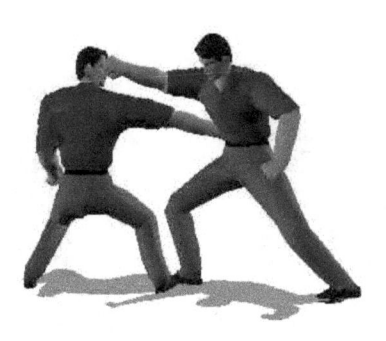

The Defender 'pop-spins' to the rear (in place) into a horse as he executes a backfist to the kidney.

There are a lot of variations for this movement in the form, but most of them are odd or advanced. You should do this part of the form extensively and keep looking at it until more applications 'pop' out at you.

APPLICATION NUMBER FOURTEEN

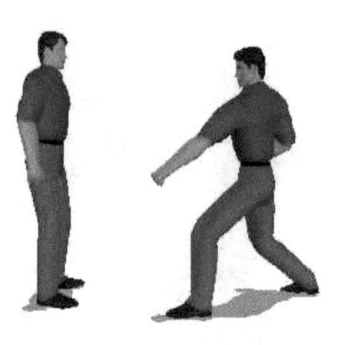

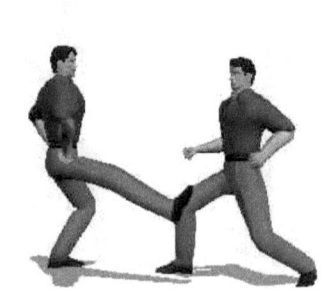

The Attacker prepares to punch.

The Attacker steps forward with the right foot into a front stance as he punches to the chest with the right hand. The Defender executes a right leg raise. This can be to the side of the knee or the groin, but for practice I like to touch the inner thigh an inch below the groin. Be gentle.

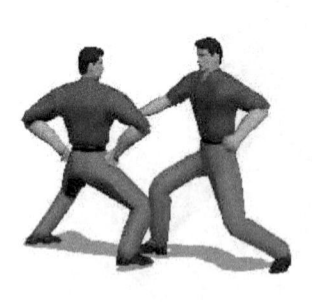

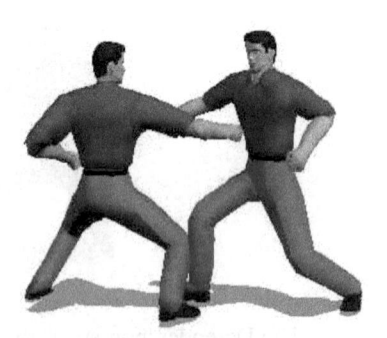

The Attacker executes a right punch. The Defender sets his right foot forward into a horse stance as he executes a right elbow block.

The Defender executes a right backfist to the rib cage. Since the Attacker's arm is extended his muscles shouldn't be able to effectively tighten, and even a soft hit can go a long way. If you wish to be precise, try for the pressure point located one inch below the nipple and one inch to the side.

APPLICATION NUMBER FIFTEEN

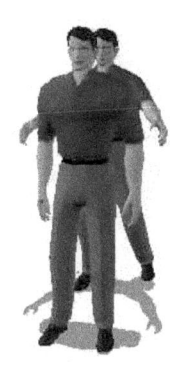

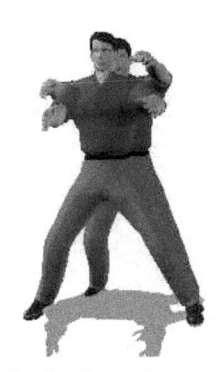

The Attacker prepares to grab the Defender from the rear.

The Defender grabs, and the Attacker steps to the right with the right foot into a horse stance as he executes a double front spear thrust to the front. This must be done at exactly the right time, the Defender must not be allowed to lock his hands. Stepping to the side exposes the Defender's centerline.

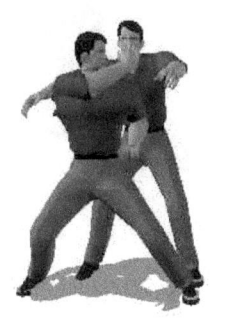

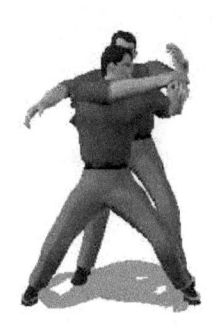

The Defender executes a right vertical elbow spike to the solar plexus and a right finger jab to the eyes.

The Defender grabs the Attacker's right arm...

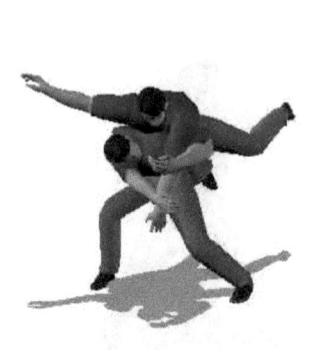

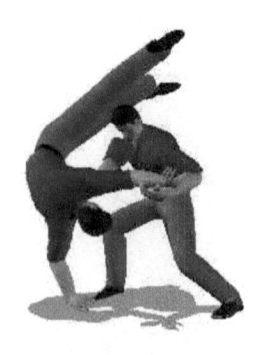

...and pivots to the left into a front stance. This will cause the Attacker to fall over the hip.

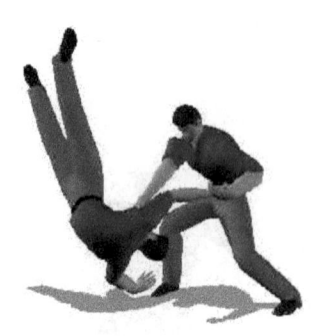

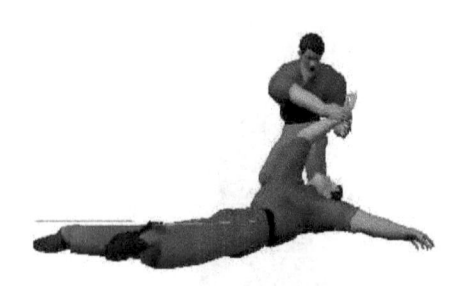

The Defender kneels, breaking the Attacker's elbow against his knee. (Don't forget to step on his face before you break his arm!)

This is a great defense with lots of variations. There are groin grabs, foot stomps and so on. If you're feeling good, step around the Attacker's arm and fall back for a classic jujitsu technique.

PINAN FOUR

The Pinans are the base of classical karate. The really neat thing about them is that they are arranged (evolved?) so that if you have a question about some point all you have to do is keep doing the form and the answer will manifest. This is sometimes difficult for beginners to understand, but as you continue to practice you will develop an intuition that will enable the form to 'speak' to you.

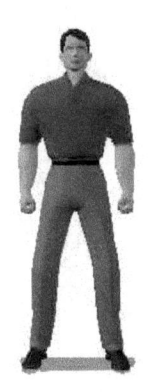

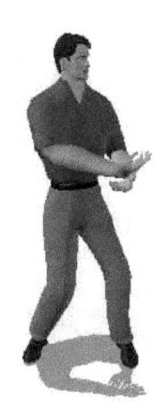

Stand in a natural stance stance. The fists should be loosely closed. The attitude and balance should be that of a person who can move instantly in any direction.
Begin pivoting to the left, scooping the hands up.

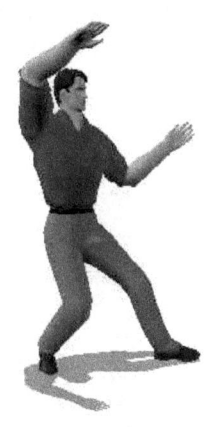

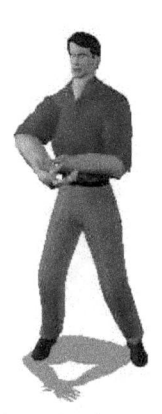

Assume a back stance as you execute a left knife block and a right high knife block. The forearms should be parallel. IT IS VERY IMPORTANT that you understand that these are two specific blocks, and not, as in some systems, a raising of the hands. As blocks, these arms align with the body and help create classical power. Why anybody ever devised the 'arm throw up' method I have no idea, for there is no power and no application to the thing.

Begin turning to the right, letting the hands continuing their motion (they did focus on the last move, but simply start them up in the same direction they were going) until they scoop in the front.

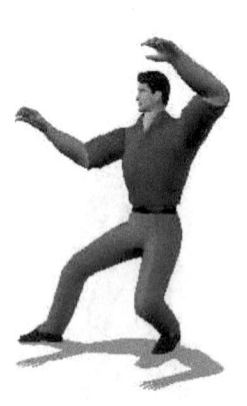

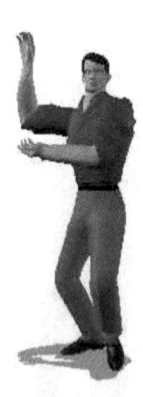

Complete the turn (180 degrees) into a back stance as you execute a right knife block and a left high knife block. Their is a subtle set up and sink of the hips, which will give you power as per the 'sand pipe visualization' mentioned in Pinan Three.

Bring the left foot up to the right and pivot to the left as you assume a back stance. The right arm should be raised so that you can achieve an effortless block by just positioning the right forearm. The left hand should scoop under the right arm. This is a good movement to show how one can catch a kick and lift it into a throw.

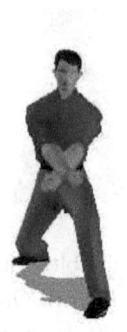

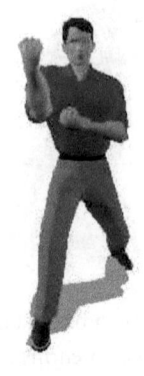

Step forward with the left foot into a front stance as you execute a low crossed wrist block. The reverse hand (the one on the opposite side of the forward foot) should be on top of the crossed wrists.

Step forward with the right foot into a front stance as a you execute a right augmented (braced or supported by the rear hand) outward middle block. This move can be done with a back stance, and even makes more sense, if one considers that the next move will require a small right foot pivot, which is more difficult with all the weight on that leg.

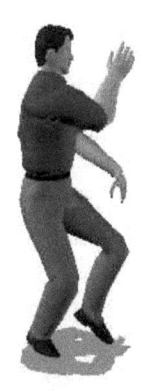

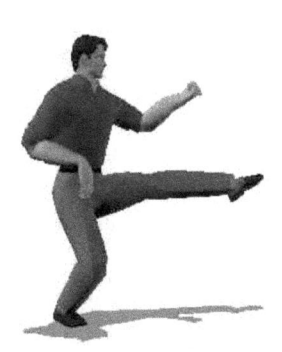

Bring the left foot forward into a cat stance as you pivot to the left and execute a left low parry and a right cross palm block.

Execute a left front snap kick and a left rolling backfist (lock it). The right arm should retract in a parry.

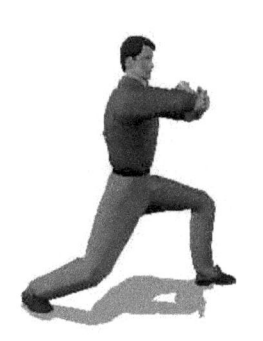

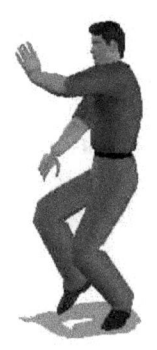

Set forward with the left foot into a front stance as you execute a right horizontal elbow. Slap the elbow with the left hand.

Bring the right foot up to the left as you pivot 180 degrees. Assume a back stance with a left cross body palm block and a right parry.

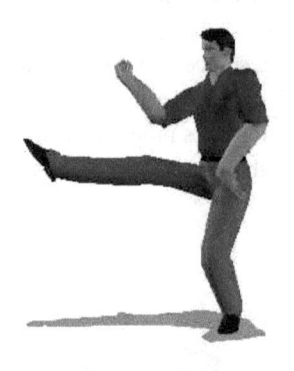

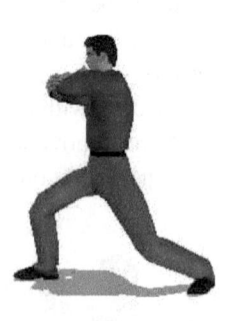

Execute a right front snap kick and a right rolling backfist (lock it). The left arm should retract in a parry.

Set forward with the right foot into a front stance as you execute a left horizontal elbow. Slap the elbow with the right hand.

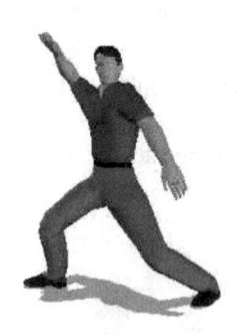

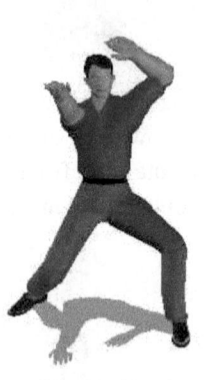

Execute a left low knife block and a right high knife block. This is a 'tiger-crane" stance. The front stance is tiger and the arms position is crane.

Pivot to the right (the front) as you execute a left high block and a right chop. The power of this technique comes form the hip twist.

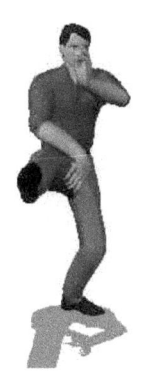

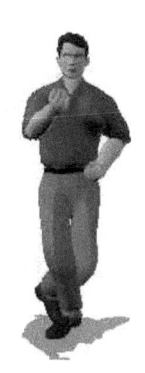

Execute a left cross palm block, a right parry, and a right front snap kick.

Place the right foot forward in an x-stance (this is like a cat stance with the toe-up foot dragged up behind the stomping foot after the stomp) as you execute a right rolling backfist. Stomping increases the weight, and therefore you have to work harder, and therefore there is more energy created, and therefore there is more energy in the movement. I often call this 'supercharging.' Make sure you do it snappy, but not so hard that you injure your stomping foot.

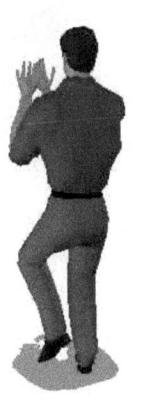

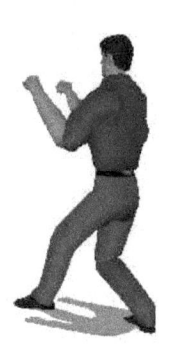

Pivot to the left 225 degrees into a cat stance as you scoop the arms down and then up in preparation for the next move.

Extend the left leg into a back stance as you execute double inverted outward middle blocks.

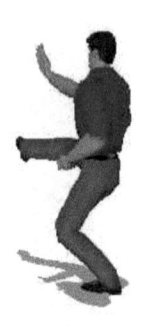

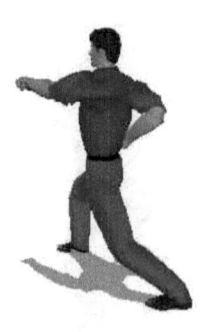

Execute a right front snap kick and a right cross palm block.
Set the right foot down in a front stance as you execute a left punch.

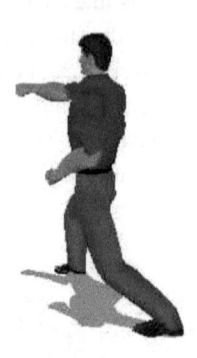

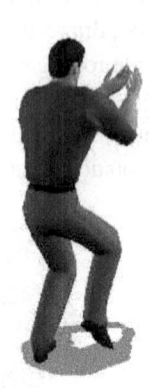

Execute a right punch. As you will see in the application, punching in this sequence ensures that you will not knock your attacker out of range with one punch.

Retract the right foot as you pivot ninety degrees to the right. Scoop the hands down and then up in preparation for the next move.

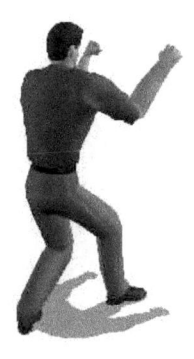

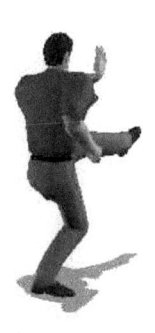

Step forward with the right foot as you execute double inverted outward middle blocks.

Execute a left front snap kick and a left cross palm block.

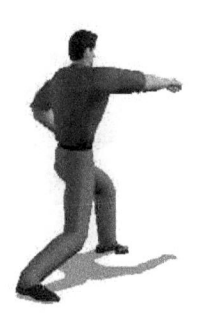

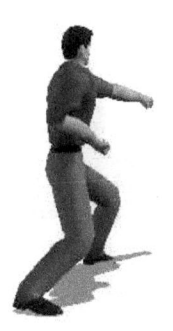

Set the left foot down in a front stance as you execute a right punch.

Execute a left punch.

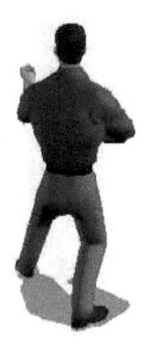

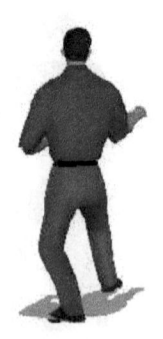

Move the left foot to the left forty-five degrees as you shift into a back stance and execute a left augmented outward middle block.

Step forward with the right foot into a back stance as you execute a right augmented outward middle block. It is possible, and advisable, to slide the blocking hand through a cross palm as you move into each of these outward blocks.

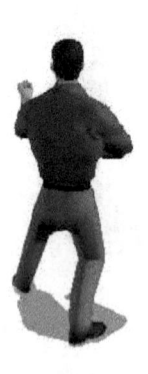

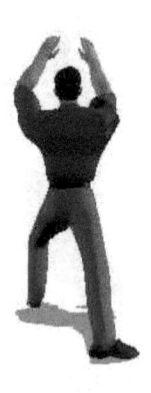

Step forward with the left foot into a back stance as you execute a left augmented outward middle block.

Step forward with the left foot as you shift into a front stance and execute double high knife blocks.

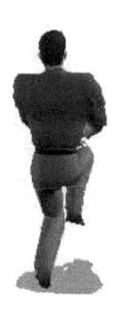

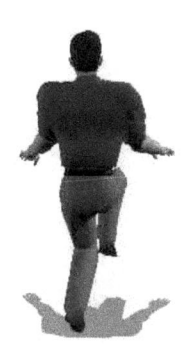

Execute a right knee strike. slap the knee with the palms of your hands and let them slide to the sides.

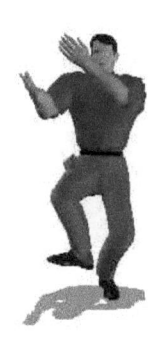

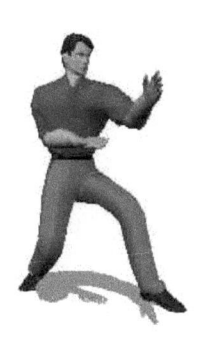

Keeping the tan tien in the same place in space, pivot 225 degrees to the left and stomp the right foot as the left foot moves outward to a back stance. The hands will go up and over to execute a left augmented knife block. This is a transitory movement that will result in a supercharge stomp.

Stomp the right foot as you assume a back stance. This will increase the weight/work/energy and supercharge the technique.

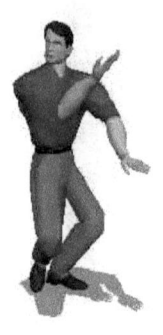

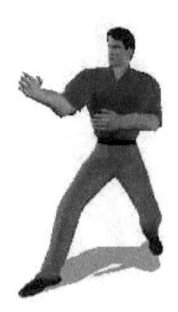

Bring the left foot back to the right foot as you prepare for a right augmented knife block.

Move the right foot out (ninety degrees from last stance) into a back stance as you execute a right augmented back stance.

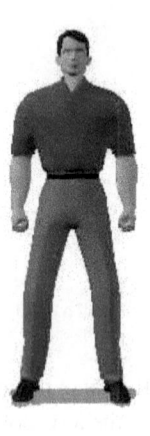

Move the right foot back and assume a natural stance to end the form.

APPLICATION NUMBER SIXTEEN

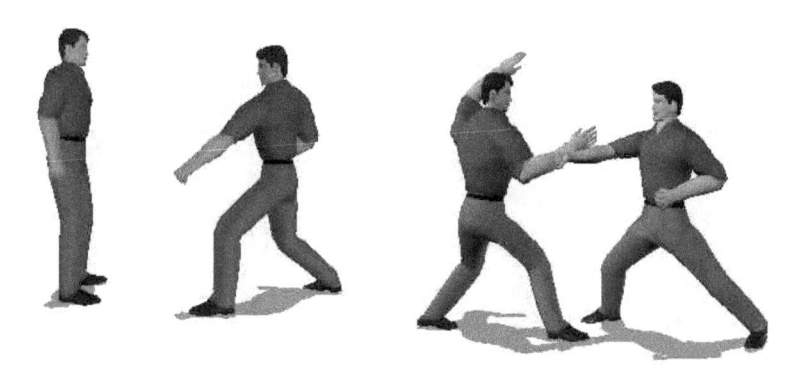

The Attacker prepares to punch.

The Attacker steps forward with the right foot into a front stance as he executes a right punch. The Defender steps back with the left foot into a back stance as he executes a right knife block and a left high knife block.

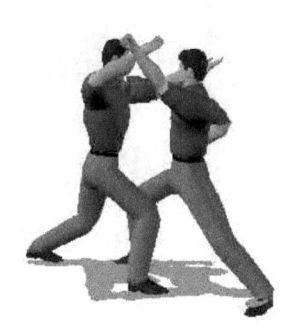

The Attacker strikes to the face with the left hand. The Defender shifts forward into a front stance as he executes a right high knife block and a left chop to the neck.

APPLICATION NUMBER SEVENTEEN

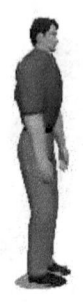

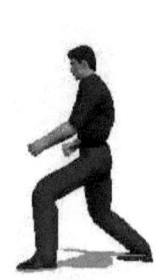

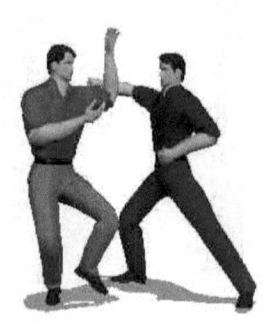

The Attacker prepares to punch.

The Attacker steps forward with the right foot as he executes a right punch to the face. The Defender assumes a cat stance as he executes a left forearm block.

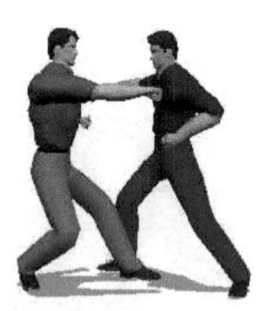

The Defender steps forward with the left foot into a back stance as he executes a right punch.

APPLICATION NUMBER EIGHTEEN

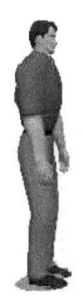

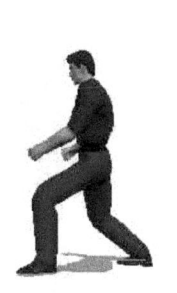

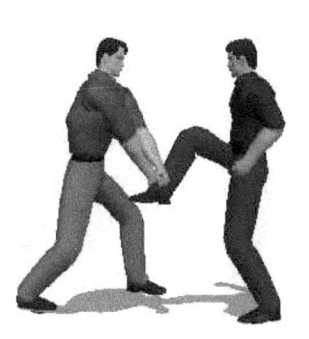

The Attacker prepares to kick.

The Attacker executes a right snap kick. The Defender moves forward with the left foot into a front stance and jams the Attacker. He executes a low crossed wrist block (right hand on top).

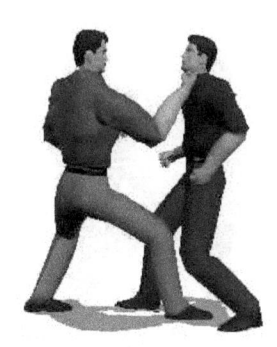

The Defender moves forward with the right foot into a back stance as he executes a right uppercut.

This application has lots of variations. One can make the uppercut into an outward block for a second punch, for instance. Examine this application, but remember that the essence of the technique is to practice it until you can move your body forward faster than he can move an arm forward.

APPLICATION NUMBER NINETEEN

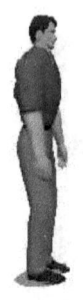

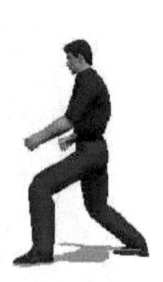

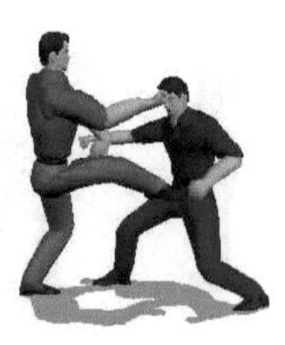

The Attacker prepares to punch.

The attacker steps forward with the right foot into a front stance as he executes a right punch. The Defender executes a left parry, a right rolling backfist, and a right snap kick to the groin.

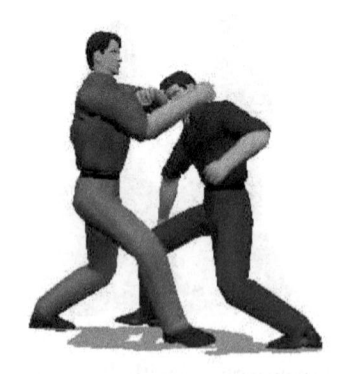

The Defender sets the right foot forward in a front stance as he grabs the head with the right hand and pulls the Attacker's head into his left horizontal elbow.

This very classical technique has lots of applications. Check out the picture below.

KANG DUK WON

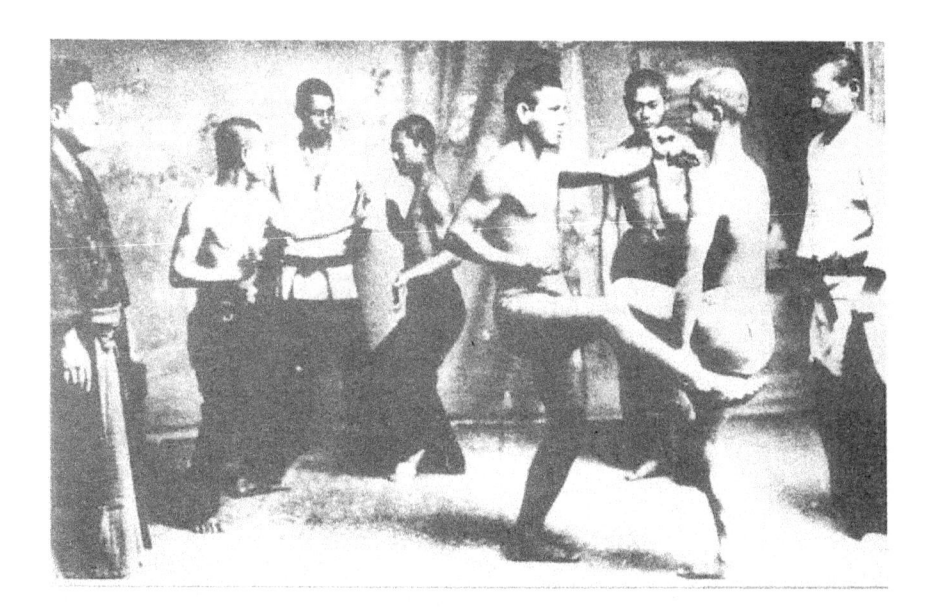

APPLICATION NUMBER TWENTY

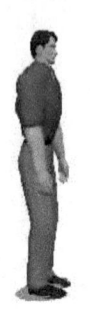

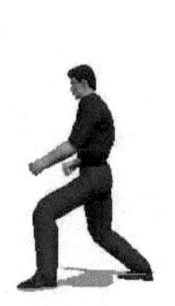

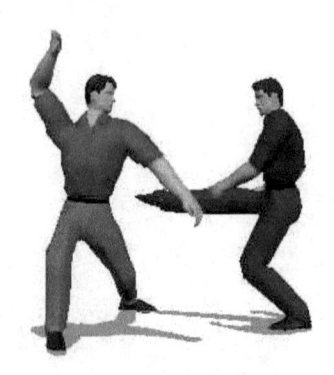

The Attacker prepares to kick.

The Attacker executes a right snap kick. The Defender steps to the right with his right foot and pivots into a front stance as he executes a right high block and a left low block.

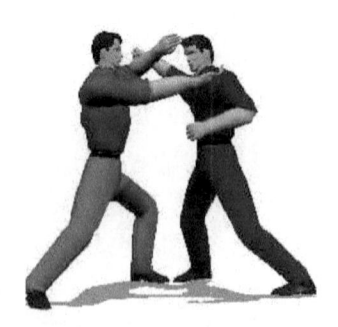

The Attacker executes a right punch to the face. The Defender pivots to the left as he executes a left high block and a right chop to the neck.

Did you ever ask yourself why you have to execute a block not being used? Like in the right high block on the first move of this technique? It is because the body must be used as a whole unit, and to not use half of it is to not use all of it. There is also the added benefit of developing proper positioning even in your preparation.

APPLICATION NUMBER TWENTY-ONE

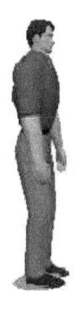

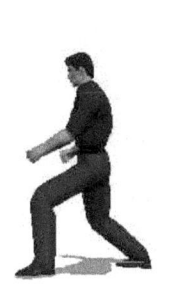

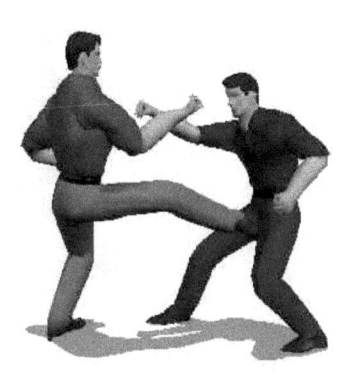

The Attacker prepares to punch.

The Attacker steps forward with the right foot into a front stance as he executes a right punch. The Defender executes a right front snap kick and a right inward middle block. Make sure the kick snaps and the block locks. The block needs to stay long enough to make sure there is no more threat from The punch, and the kick must not hang out in space waiting to be grabbed.

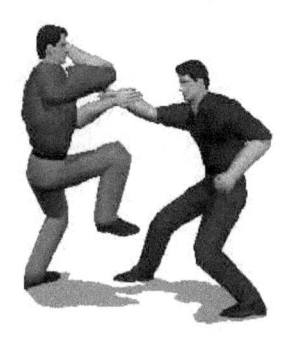

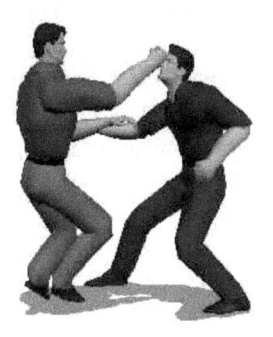

The Defender grabs the Attacker's right arm with his left hand. The Defender's left hand must go outside his right hand, else there will be a potential, from slight forward push by the Attacker, for the Defender's hands to be trapped. The right hand prepares for a vertical backfist.

The Defender executes a stomping right foot into an X-stance (the left foot is pulled up behind right after) as he pulls the Attacker's right arm and executes a right vertical backfist to the bridge of the nose.

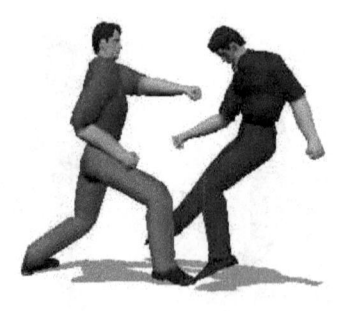

The Defender steps forward with the right foot into a front stance and executes a the mother of all left punches.

A couple of interesting points:

One, stomping, by increasing the weight=work=energy, will supercharge a technique, and this is valuable for creating a strong backfist, which is not usually a strong technique.

Two, and this leads us to this **MAJOR HINT**:

Create a LINE to your opponent with your technique, but MAKE SURE YOUR BODY IS SOLIDLY BEHIND THE LINE! If you don't, then you are striking with an arm's worth of weight, instead of your whole body weight.

APPLICATION NUMBER TWENTY-TWO

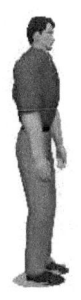

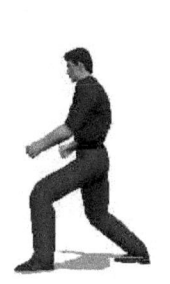

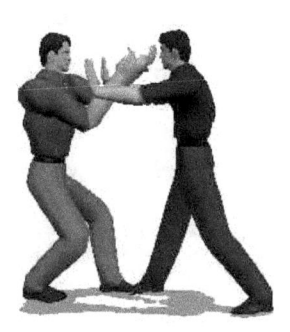

The Attacker prepares to push to the chest with both hands.

The Attacker steps forward with the right foot into a front stance as he executes a double handed push to the chest. The Defender begins moving his right leg back and raises his forearms in between the Attacker's arms.

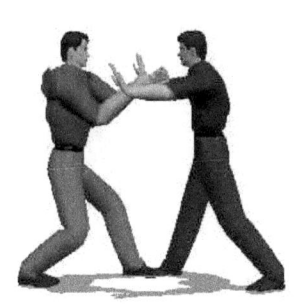

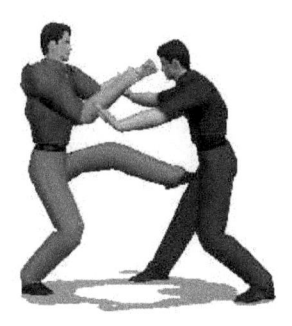

The Defender sets his right foot down in a back stance as he executes double inverted outward middle blocks.

The Defender executes a left front snap kick to the groin.

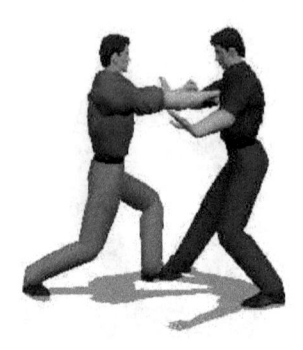

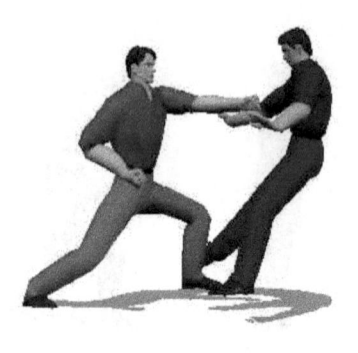

The Defender sets the left foot into a front stance as he executes a right punch.

The Defender pivots slightly to the left as he executes a left punch.

If you punch with the wrong hand first the Attacker might be thrust out of range of the next punch. Make sure you use the right amount of hip power on each punch.

APPLICATION NUMBER TWENTY-THREE

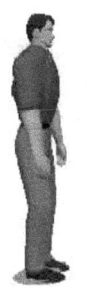

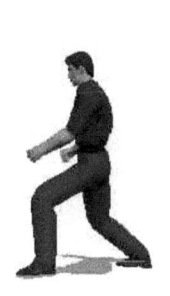

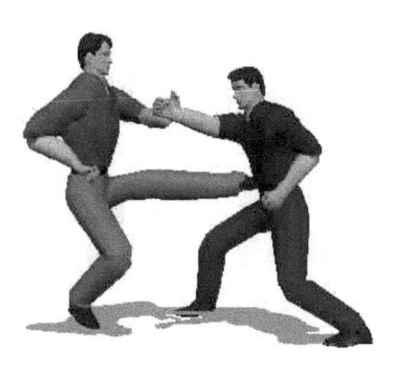

The Attacker prepares to punch.

The Attacker steps forward with the right foot into a front stance as he executes a right punch. The Defender executes a left snap kick and a left cross palm block.

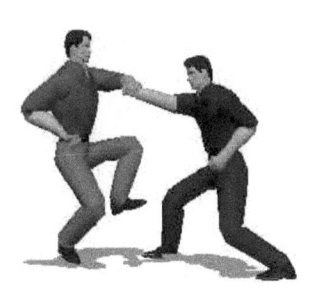

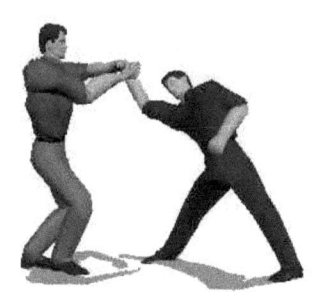

The Defender retracts the left leg as he reaches over and grips the Attacker's right fist with his left hand.

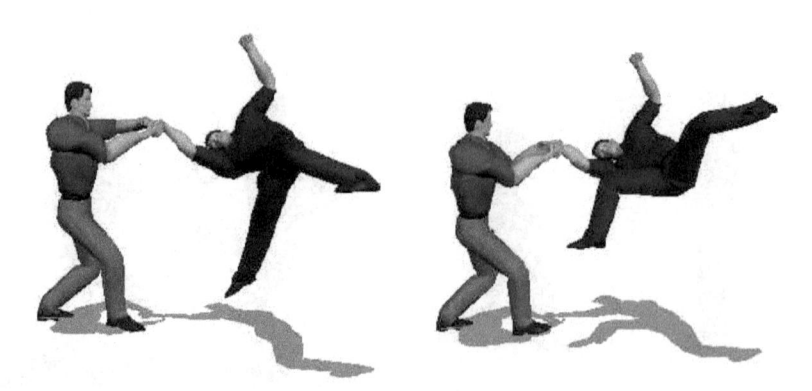

The Defender keeps moving back with the left leg to a back stance as he turns the Attacker's wrist over.

Isn't this a nice one?

Striking (as in the kick) is helpful when one wants to make a grab art (in this case a wrist lock) work. This is called 'Shock and Lock.'

Of course, when practicing this with a friend, you might wish to be slow and gentle with the wrist lock and let him turn backwards and do a back roll.

APPLICATION NUMBER TWENTY-FOUR

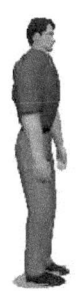

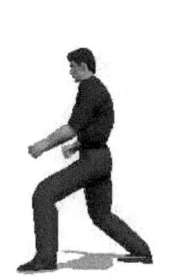

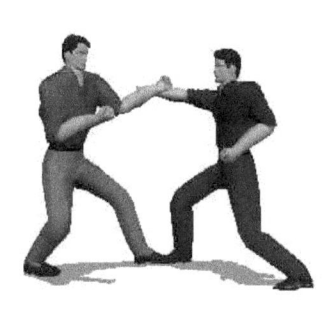

The Attacker prepares to punch.

The Attacker steps forward with the right foot as he executes a right punch. The Defender steps back with the left foot into a back stance as he executes a left outward middle block.

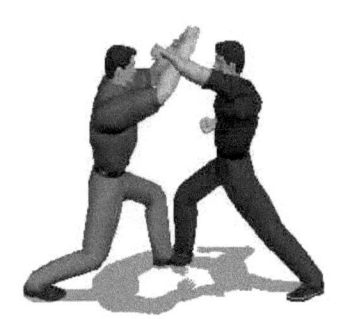

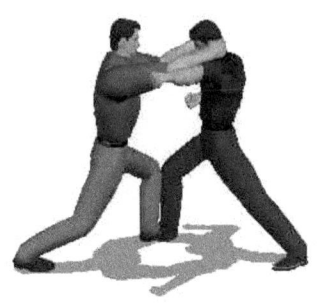

The Defender executes a left punch to the face. The Defender shifts forward into a front stance as he executes double high knife blocks.

The Defender grabs the Attacker around the neck.

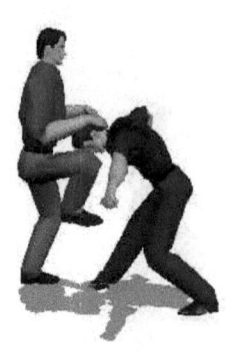

The Defender pulls the Attacker's head down as he executes a right knee to the face.

PINAN FIVE

The Pinans are the base of classical karate. The really neat thing about them is that they are arranged (evolved?) so that if you have a question about some point all you have to do is keep doing the form and the answer will manifest. This is sometimes difficult for beginners to understand, but as you continue to practice you will develop an intuition that will enable the form to 'speak' to you.

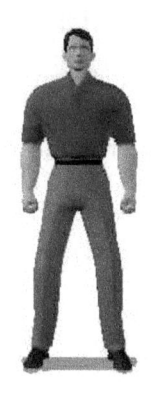

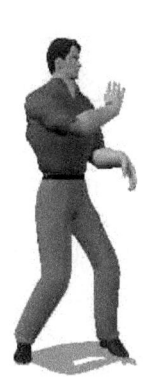

Standing in the natural stance.

Turn to the left as you execute a right cross palm block. The left hand raises slightly in a parry.

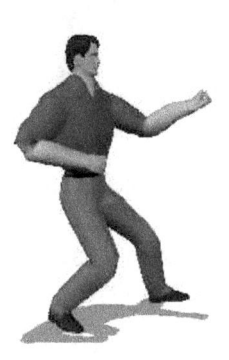

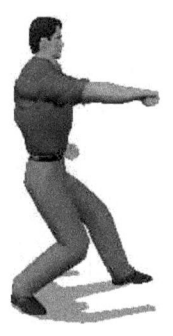

Assume a back stance as you execute a left outward middle block. There is subtle hip shifting in this sequence of movements. Examine them carefully, and make sure the body is properly aligned.

Execute a right punch.

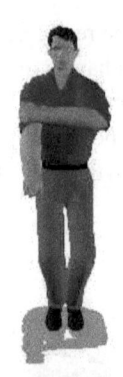

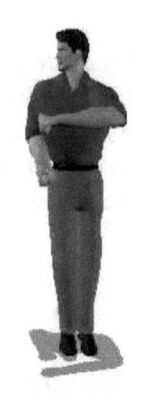

Bring the right foot up to the left foot as you turn ninety degrees to the front. Your right arm should stay extended, as if part of the body, when you turn. Your legs are bent.

Straighten up slowly, retracting the right hand and turning the head to the right.

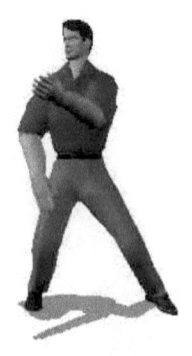

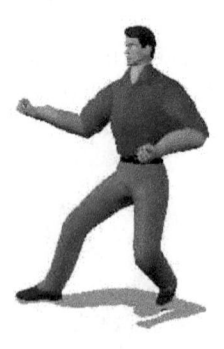

Turn to the right as you execute a left cross palm block. The right hand raises slightly in a parry.

Assume a back stance as you execute a right outward middle block. There is subtle hip shifting in this sequence of movements. Examine them carefully, and make sure the body is properly aligned.

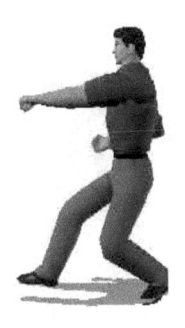

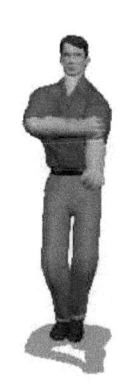

Execute a left punch.

Bring the left foot up to the right foot as you turn ninety degrees to the front. Your left arm should stay extended, as if part of the body, when you turn. Your legs are bent.

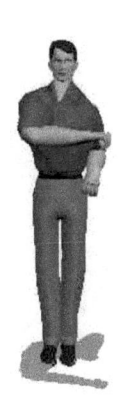

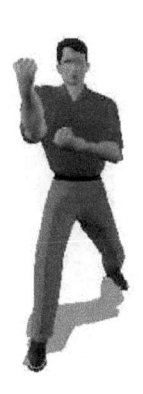

Straighten up slowly, retracting the right hand and facing to the front.

Step forward with the right foot into a front stance as you execute a left augmented outward middle block.

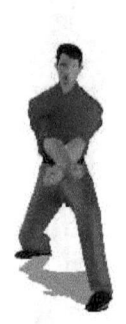

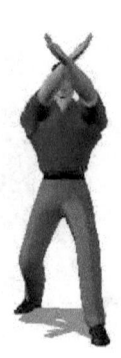

Step forward with the left foot into a front stance as you execute a low crossed wrist block.

Shift back into a back stance as you execute a high crossed wrist knife hand block.

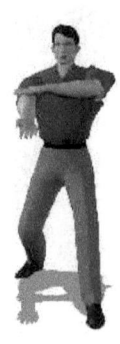

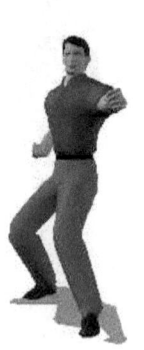

Turn the palms so that they face each other, then circle the hands until the left hand is over the right elbow, and the right hand is extended to the front.

Execute a left backfist. Make sure you add a subtle hip motion to this move so that the body stays aligned.

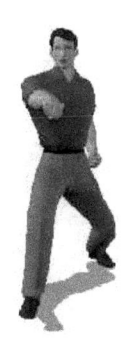

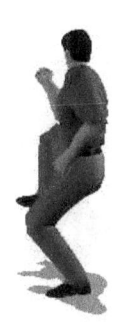

Step forward with the right foot into a front stance as you execute a right punch.

Swing the right knee and a right inward block to the left, all the way to the rear.

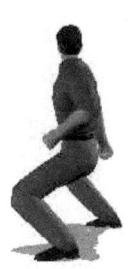

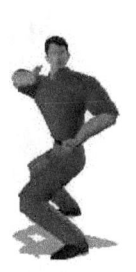

Stomp the right foot into a horse stance as you execute a right low block.

Swing the right hand back to the front in an open hand block with the fingers pointing horizontal.

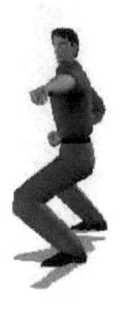

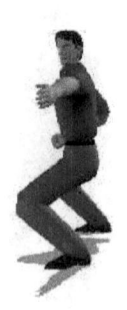

Retract the right hand as you execute a left punch.
Turn the left palm and open it.

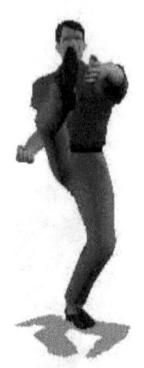

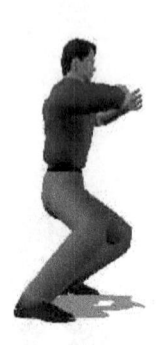

Execute a right crescent kick to your left palm.
Set the right foot down in the horse stance as you execute a right horizontal elbow strike to your left palm.

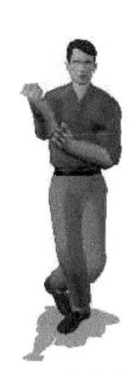

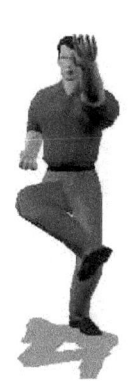

Bring your left foot up behind your right foot as you assume an x-stance. Execute a right augmented outward middle block.

Shift your weight to the right foot as you raise the left knee (the foot can be turned as in a low crescent block). Retract the right hand as you execute a left spear hand.

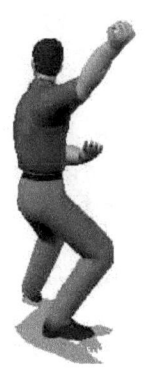

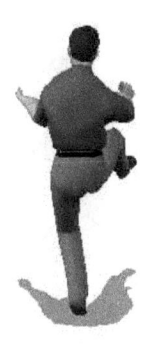

Stomp the right foot (similar to the stomp near the beginning of Pinan Two) as you pivot to the rear in a back stance. Execute a right inverted upward thrusting punch. the left hand should be available to guard the body under the punching arm.

Swing the right foot and the arms upward.

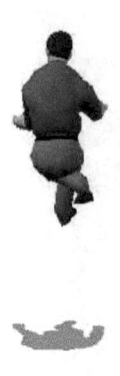

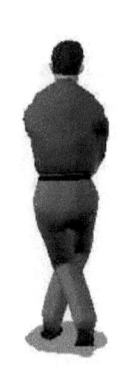

As you leap, bring the left foot up tight.

Land in an x-stance with a low crossed wrist block. The right arm should be on top.

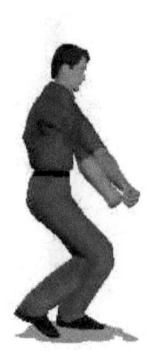

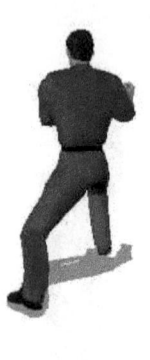

Here is a side view of the previous photo.

Step forward with the right foot into a front stance as you execute an augmented right outward middle block.

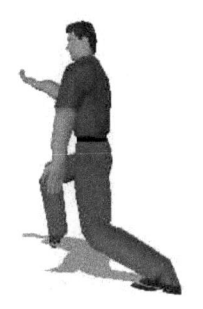

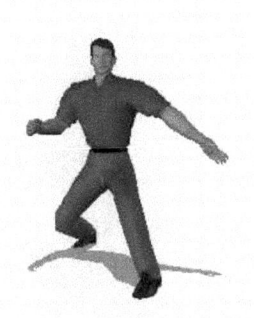

Move the rear foot behind yourself (to the left) so you will be able to pivot and face in the opposite direction in a front stance with the feet shoulders width apart. Swing the left arm down in an inverted low block to cover the groin.

Pivot, circling the left hand up for the cross palm block and starting to shoot the right hand towards the spear.

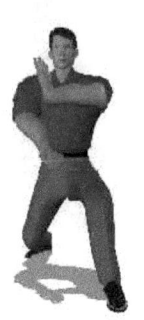

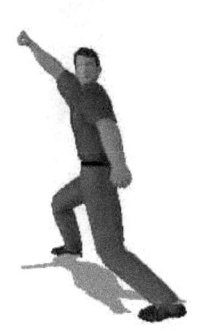

Assuming a front stance with the left foot forward, execute a right spear to the groin and a left palm block.

Pivot to the right into a front stance as you execute a right low block and a left (shoulder high) outward middle block.

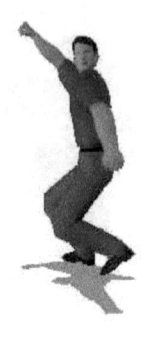

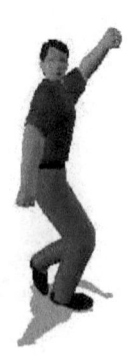

Bring the left foot back and place it next to the right foot.

Pivot in place into an x-stance as you execute a right low block and a left (shoulder high) outward middle block.

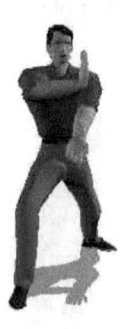

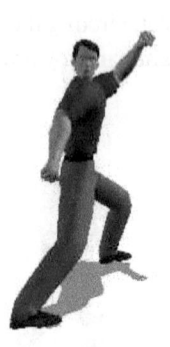

Step forward with the right foot into a front stance as you execute a left spear to the groin and a right cross palm block.

Pivot to the left into a front stance as you execute a left low block and a right (shoulder high) outward middle block.

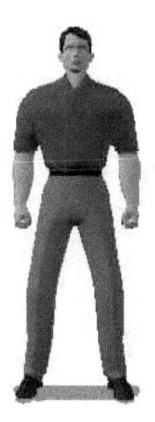

Step forward with the left foot and assume a natural stance.

APPLICATION NUMBER TWENTY-FIVE

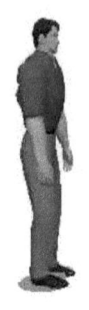

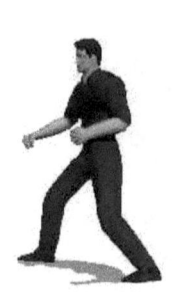

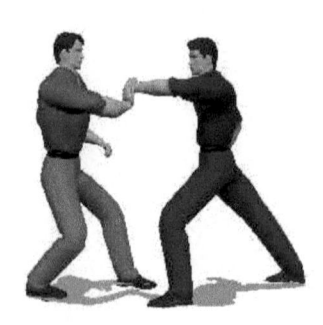

The Attacker prepares to punch.

The Attacker steps forward with the left leg into a front stance as he punches to the face with the right hand. The Defender steps back with the right foot into a back stance as he executes a right cross palm block.

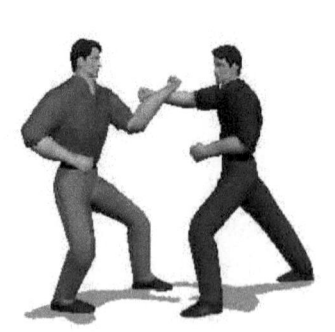

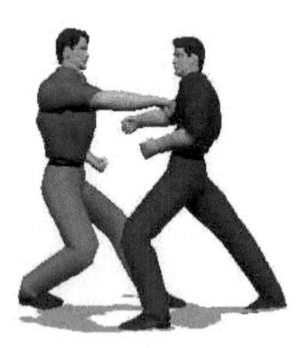

The Attacker executes a right punch. The Defender executes a left outward middle block.

The Defender executes a right punch.

While this looks like a common blocking pattern, the essence is on looking 'liquid.' don't focus so much as slide through. By this time the student should have lots of power, now he has to make it look smooth. And he has to fit the action into smaller and smaller spaces.

Interestingly, good karate is whiplike. It looks more like Tai Chi, at the upper reaches, than karate.

APPLICATION NUMBER TWENTY-SIX

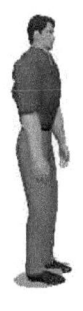

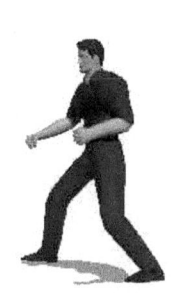

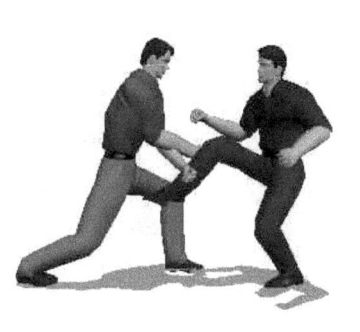

The Attacker prepares to kick.

The Attacker executes a right snap kick. The Defender moves forward, jamming the Attacker (jamming the kick before the power comes out), as he executes a low crossed wrist block.

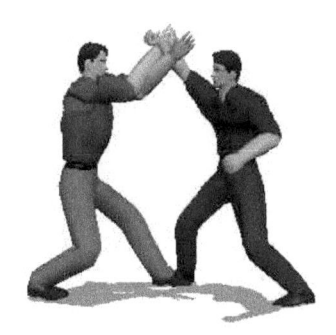

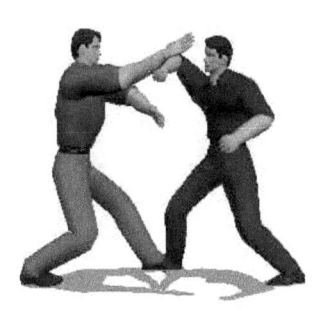

The Attacker sets the right foot down into a front stance and, seeing that the Defender is leaning forward, executes a strike the face. The Defender shifts back into a back stance as he executes a high crossed wrist block.

The Defender moves the right hand in a circle, sweeping the Attacker's right arm around and out, thus exposing the chest.

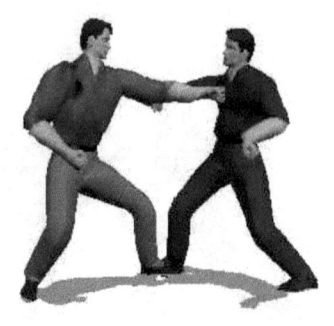

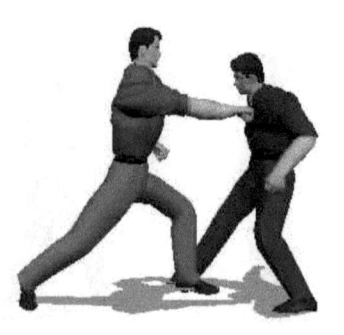

The Defender executes a left backfist to the chest.

The Defender executes a right punch to the chest. Though I have showed this technique with a front stance, it should be done with a back stance, shuffling forward if distance needs to be covered.

This technique has a *lot* of variations. It is great for club disarms, armbars, blocks for secondary attacks, necklocks, and so on.

APPLICATION NUMBER TWENTY-SEVEN

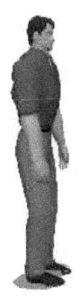

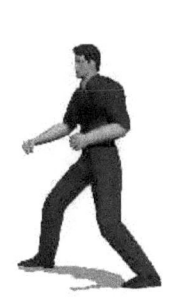

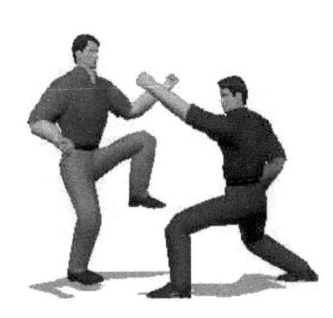

The Attacker prepares to punch.

The Attacker steps forward with the left foot into a front stance as he executes a left punch. The Defender executes a left inward middle block as he brings the left knee up.

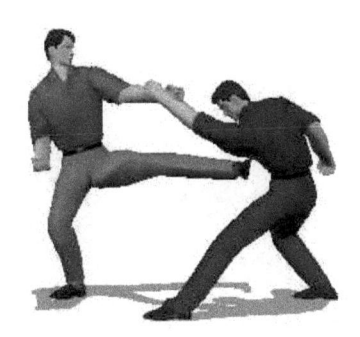

The Defender executes a left side thrust kick. If possible, pull the Attacker's arm so as to stop him from blocking or running.

This can also be used to block a kick, followed by a counter with a backfist.

APPLICATION NUMBER TWENTY-EIGHT

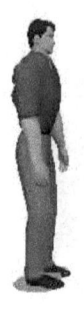

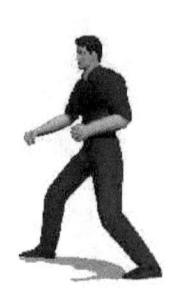

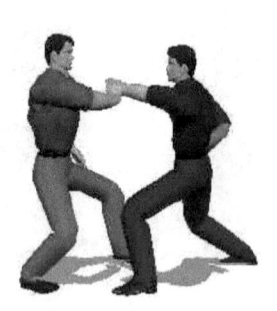

The Attacker prepares to punch.

The Attacker steps forward with the left foot into a front stance as he executes a left punch. The Defender steps back with the right foot into a back stance as he executes a right cross palm block.

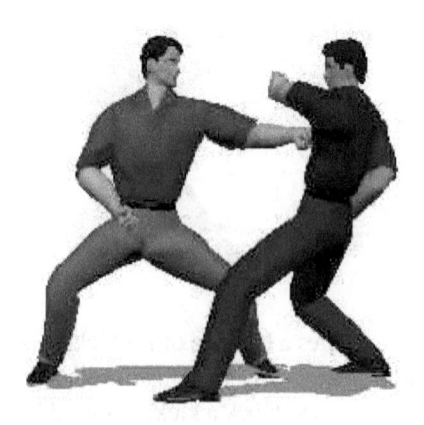

The Defender pivots (which includes dropping the weight greatly) into a horse stance as he executes a left punch to the axilla (nerve center in the armpit.

I call this the Horse Punch, or The Power Punch.

APPLICATION NUMBER TWENTY-NINE

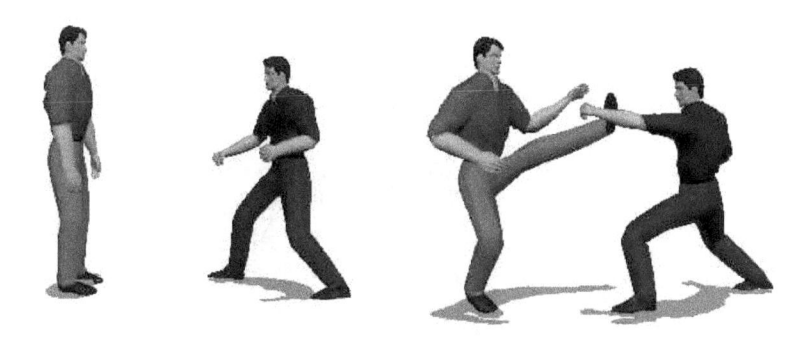

The Attacker prepares to punch.

The Attacker steps forward with the left foot into a front stance as he executes a left punch. The Defender executes a left crescent kick to the Attacker's fist.

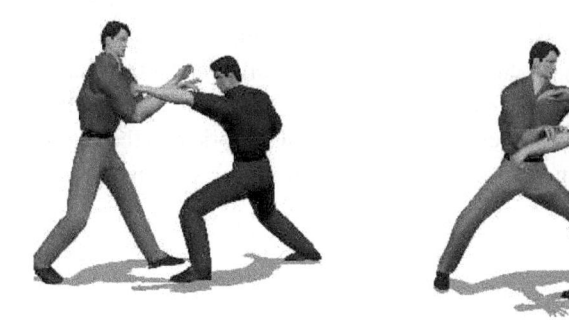

The Defender moves forward as he grips the Attacker's arm.

The Defender assumes a horse stance as he pulls the Attacker forward and executes a left elbow to the face.

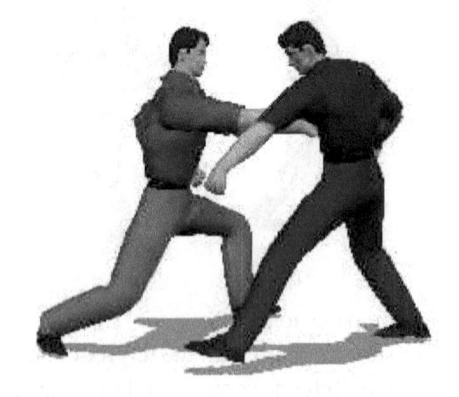

The Defender pivots to the left as he executes a right punch.

The idea, here, is that the feet must be as quick as the hands. (And the hands must be as powerful as the feet.) This technique *can* be done. If you can't do it now, then simply practice it until you can. Really, one of the secrets of karate is that if you can make the large motion of the classical technique work, then you can make the shortened street version also work, and the shortened street version will then have classical power in it. I can't say anything more than that.

APPLICATION NUMBER THIRTY

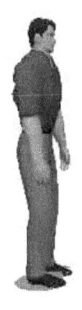

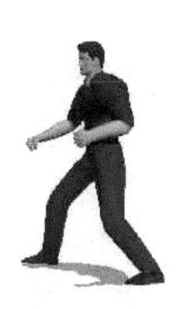

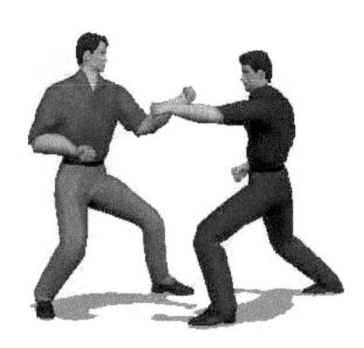

The Attacker prepares to punch.

The Attacker steps forward with the left foot into a front stance as he executes a left punch. The Defender steps back with the right foot into a back stance as he executes a left inward middle block.

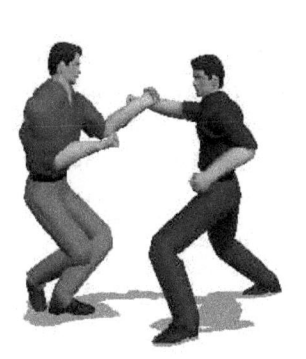

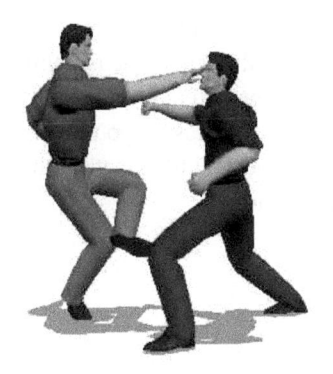

The Attacker executes a right punch. The Defender moves the right foot forward and behind the left foot in an x-stance as he executes a left augmented outward middle block.

The Attacker lifts the left foot in a sole block (assuming a crane stance) as he retracts the left hand and executes a right spear to the eyes. The raised foot could be a knee knocker, but it's really just to prepare for the supercharging footstomp.

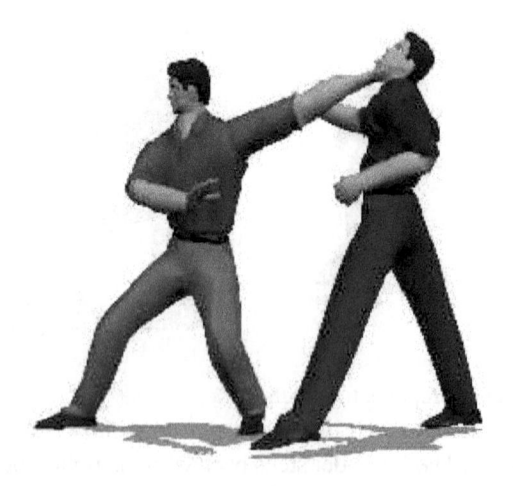

The Attacker stomps the foot (supercharging weight/work/energy) as he pivots 180 degrees and executes a left thrusting uppercut. The right hand guards the body under the thrusting uppercut.

Obviously, one is training for the eventuality of somebody trying to sneak up behind him. But the real idea here is to train yourself to move the whole body as fast as your opponent can move an arm. If this isn't obvious to you with just a little practice, then you should go back and practice the earlier applications.

APPLICATION NUMBER THIRTY-ONE

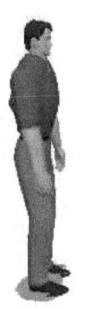

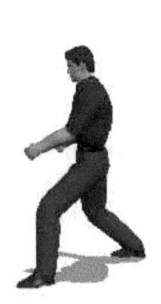

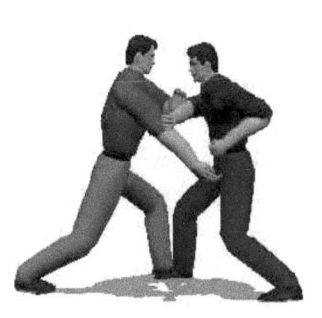

The Attacker prepares to punch.

The Attacker steps forward with the right foot into a front stance as he executes a right punch. The Defender steps forward with the left foot into a front stance as he executes a left cross palm block and a right spear to the groin.

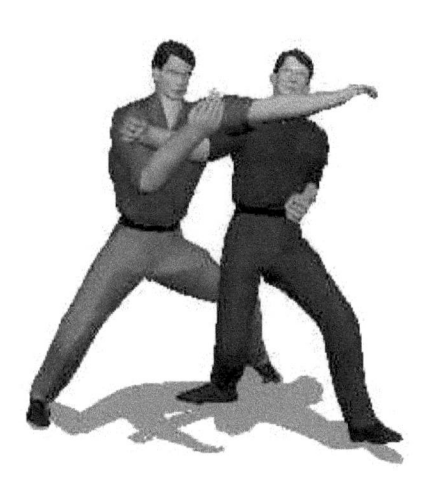

The Defender pivots into a horse stance (he might have to shuffle further behind the Attacker to make this work) as he traps the Attacker's right arm with his right arm and shoots his left arm across the Attacker's neck.

This technique is called 'splitting.' The Attacker's lower body goes forward and the upper body goes backward. This is a great technique, very workable, and there are lots of great variations. If one followed the classic move of the form he could simply break the shoulder with the elbow as he slaps the groin. And a punch could be added on the end. And so on and so on. Do it a lot and all of the techniques will become very apparent.

It is said, which might mean this is just rumor...but there might be a glint of truth in it, too...that Gichin Funakoshi (the 'George Washington' of Karate) took a few lessons from Jigoro Kano (the founder of Judo). At one point Funakoshi is said to have worked a throw, and Jigoro said, 'I didn't show you that.' Funakoshi merely replied that there were throws in karate.

I like this story, because I believe there is truth in it. There are throws in karate, lots of them. And, to be truthful, when karate was exported through Japan it picked up a military mindset which seemed more concerned with training masses to specialize in the strikes for which karate is known for. So...who knows.

At any rate, practice throws like the one above, and practice them a lot.

APPLICATION NUMBER THIRTY-TWO

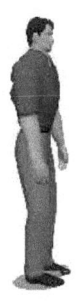

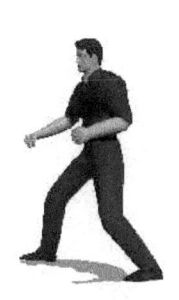

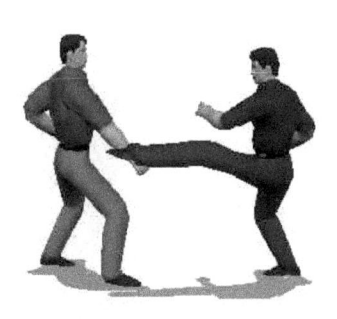

The Attacker prepares to kick.

The Attacker executes a left kick. The Defender steps back with the right foot into a back stance as he executes a right low block.

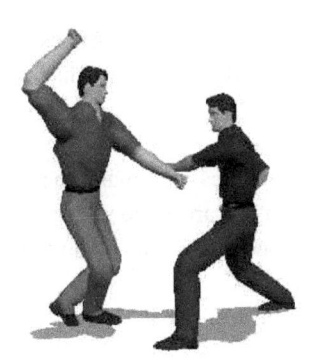

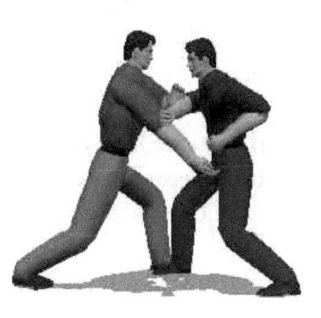

The Attacker executes a left punch to the body. The Defender retracts the left foot and twists into an x-stance as he executes a right low block and a left high block.

The Attacker executes a right punch to the face. The Defender steps forward with the left foot into a front stance as he executes a left cross palm block and continues the circling motion of the high block back and around and into a right spear to the groin.

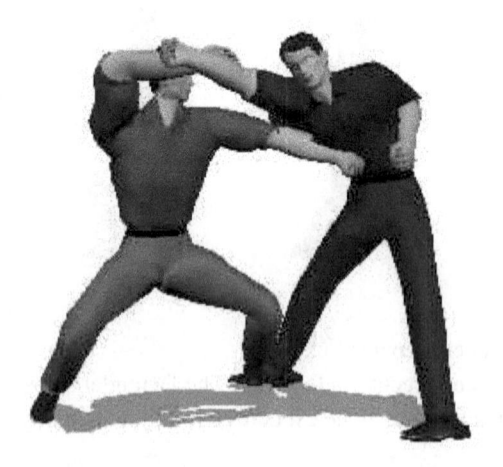

The Defender pivots into a horse stance as he grabs the Attacker's right arm with his right arm and executes a high block and a left hammerfist to the solar plexus.

If you ever have trouble with a technique, break it down into pieces and practice those pieces until they are fast enough to be part of the whole technique. Compare applications thirty-one and thirty-two and this should be obvious.

Add a downward punch at the end, if you feel like it.

SIPSU

This next block of forms, Sipsu, Nohai, Botsai, Umbe, and The Iron Horse, are considered brown belt forms in many systems. Having done the Pinans, one should be very competent in basics, and these forms begin the process of developing internal power.

I have spelled the names phonetically, for the most part, because there is usually some disagreement as to exact name and pronunciation. Interestingly, the names are specific to the arts, and often people who speak the language don't even know what they mean. Sipsu is supposed to mean 'ten hands.'

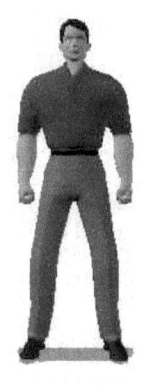

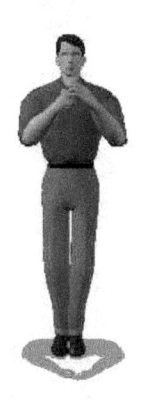

Start in the natural stance.
Pull the right foot in and raise the hands so that the right fist is cupped by the left hand. this hand configuration is supposed to mean I have a weapon, but it is still in the sheath.

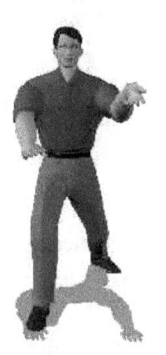

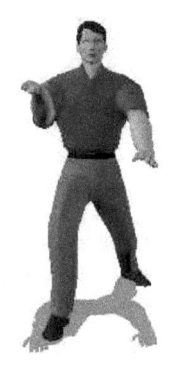

Shoot the left foot back, assuming a front stance, as you execute a right palmdown block and a left palm up block. Make sure the hands are parallel to the ground.

Execute a left palm down block and a right palm up block. Do this with great tension, as if you are moving thousands of pounds. Make sure you breath deeply and put 110% into the movement.

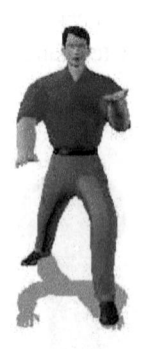

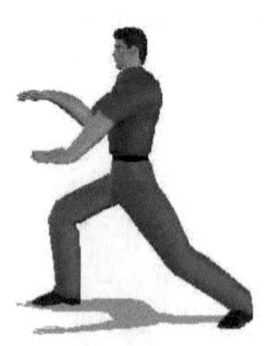

Step forward with the left foot into a front stance as you execute a left palm up block and a right palm down block.

Step forward with the right foot and then to the right into a front stance as you execute a right palm up block and a left palm down block.

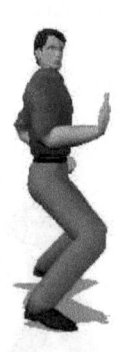

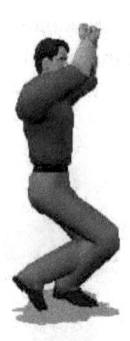

Step to the left with the right foot into a horse stance as you execute a right palm block at waist level. There can be two more of these moving forward in the form, but I prefer to do just one.

Move the right foot in front of the left foot in an x-stance as you execute a high crossed wrist block.

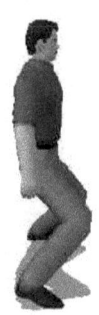

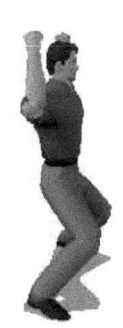

Move the left foot to the left as you execute double low blocks to the sides.

Jump to the left into a horse stance as you execute double shoulder high outward blocks.

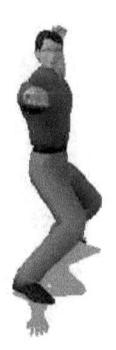

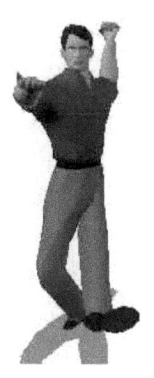

Extend the right arm to the right as you look to the right.
Execute a left oblique foot stomp to the right.

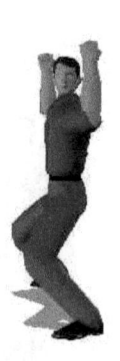

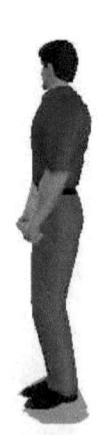

Set the left foot down in a horse stance as you snap the arms around to execute a right shoulder high outward block and a left shoulder high inward block.

There can be two more of these last movements, but I prefer doing a shorter form with just one.

Bring the right foot next to the left foot as you stand up and look to the right. the fist should be in front of your thighs.

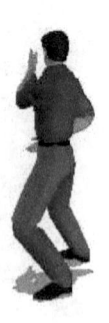

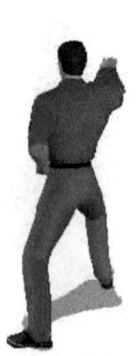

Step to the left as you prepare the right hand for a chop and protect the face with a left palm block.

Assume a front stance as you execute a right chop.

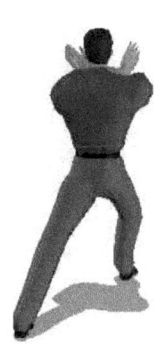

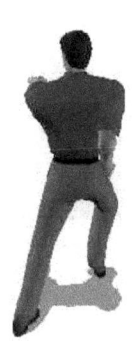

Twist to the right as you prepare the left hand for a chop. The right hand protects the face.

Assume a twisted stance as you execute a left chop

Can you find an application for this last sequence of moves?

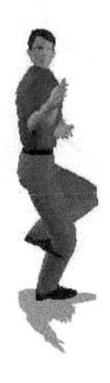

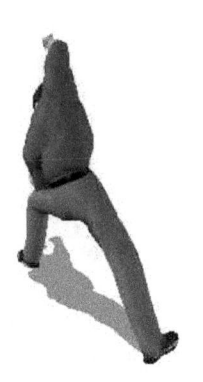

Circle the hands over and down as you assume a crane stance (left foot hooked behind the knee) and execute a right knife block.

Step to the left into a front stance as you execute a left punch to the groin and a right punch to the face. I call this an over/under punch. The forearms must be parallel, and the fists and the head must be as if striking the target simultaneously. (Go up to a wall and touch your fists and head simultaneously to the wall to see what I mean.)

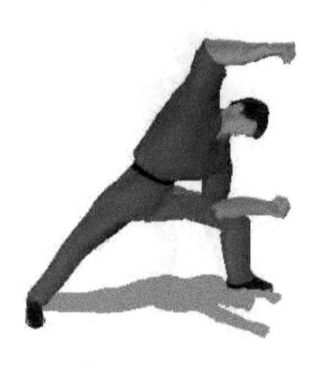

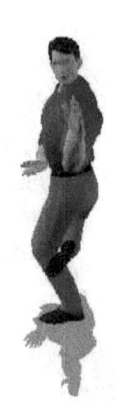

Here is a side view of the previous move.
Hook the right foot behind the left knee in a crane as you bring the hands over to a knife block.

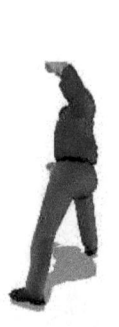

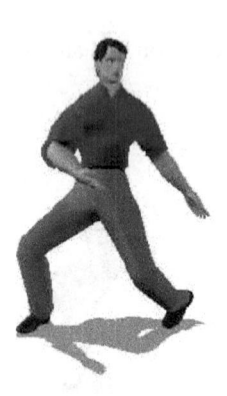

Step forward with the right foot into a front stance as you execute an over/under punch. (Left to face and right to groin.)
Move the left foot to the right, behind your right foot, swinging the right arm down to cover the groin.

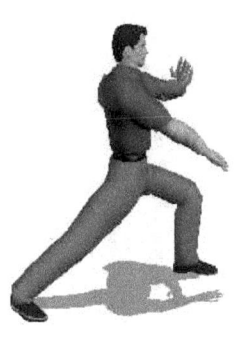

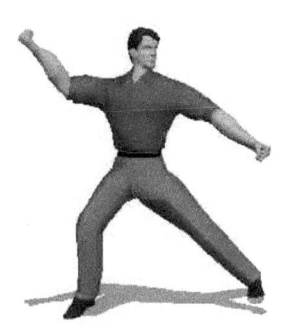

Move into a front stance as you execute a left cross palm block and a right spear to the groin.

Pivot to the right and assume a front stance in the other direction as you execute a left hammer to the groin and a right shoulder high outward block.

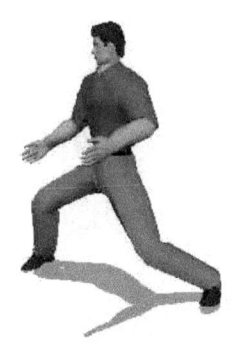

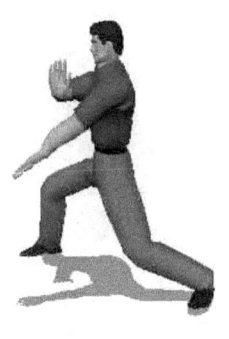

Stump the right leg behind yourself so that you can face squarely in the other direction. Move the right arm down to to cover the groin as you circle into the next move.

Assume a front stance as you execute a right cross palm and a left spear to the groin.

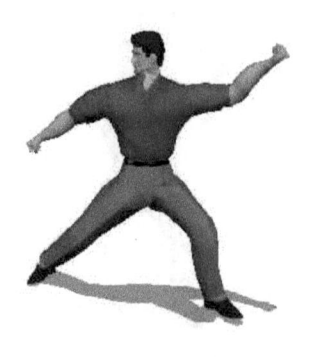

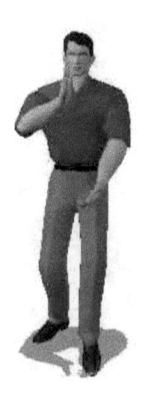

Pivot to the left into a front stance as you execute a right low block to the groin and a left shoulder high outward block.

Bring the left foot into a cat stance and face to the right (forward in the form) as you protect the face with a right cross palm block and a left scoop at the groin level.

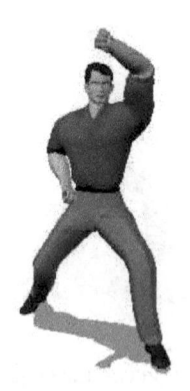

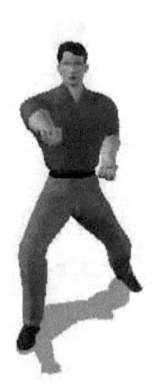

Step forward with the left foot into a front stance as you execute a left high block.

Step forward with the right foot into a front stance as you execute a right punch.

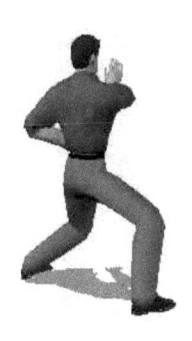

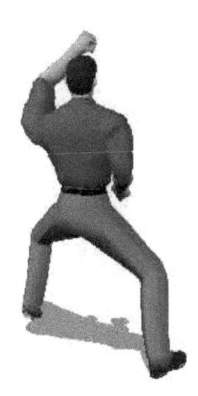

Stump the left foot behind yourself so that you can face squarely to the rear. As you do so protect the face with a right cross palm block. The left hand scoops and begins coming up the centerline for a high block.

Assume a front stance to the rear as you execute a left high block.

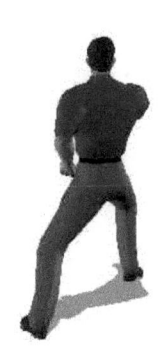

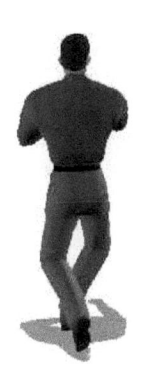

Step forward with the right foot into a front stance as you execute a right punch.

Bring the left foot up to the back of the right (toes to heel) and prepare to turn into the next position.

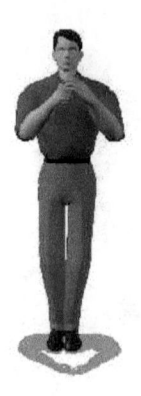

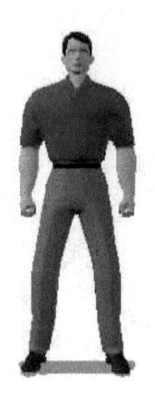

Pivot in place and assume the beginning posture.
Return to the natural stance.

APPLICATION NUMBER THIRTY-THREE

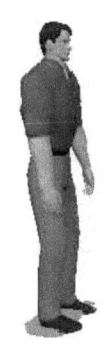

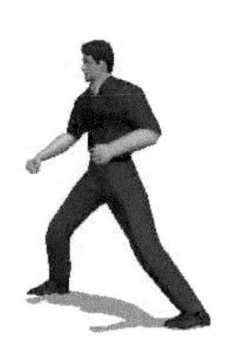

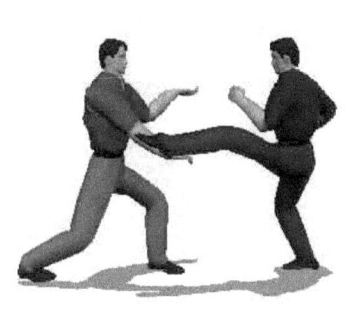

The Attacker prepares to punch.

The Attacker executes a left snap kick. The Defender steps back with the right foot into a front stance as he executes a left palm up block and a right palm down block.

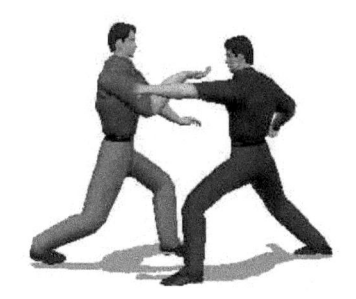

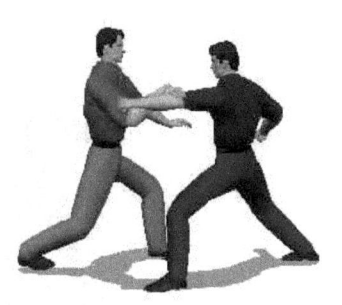

The Attacker sets forward in a front stance as he executes a left punch. The Defender executes a left palm down block and a right palm up block.

The Defender turns his right hand over to hook the attacker's arm.

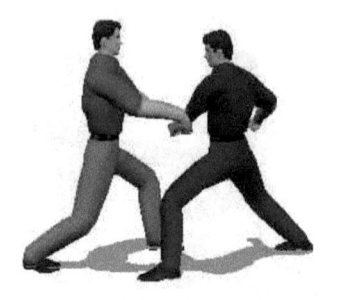

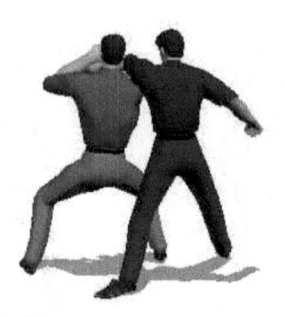

The Defender starts circling the Attacker's arm down and across his body. If there is resistance simply step with the whole body.

The Defender steps forward and in front of the Attacker with his right foot into a horse stance as he places the Attacker's arm across his shoulder. The contact point should be the Attacker's elbow. A quick pull down and the Attacker's elbow is broken. One can step further and circle further to create Aikido style throws, etc. Variations depend upon body distancing and joints selected.

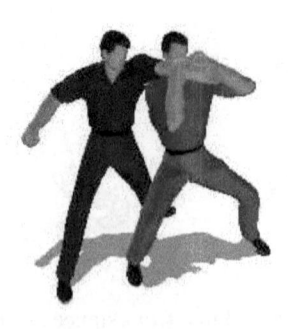

Here's a view from the other side.

The secret of understanding forms is learning how to examine them for variations. You'll understand this more after doing the next application.

APPLICATION NUMBER THIRTY-FOUR

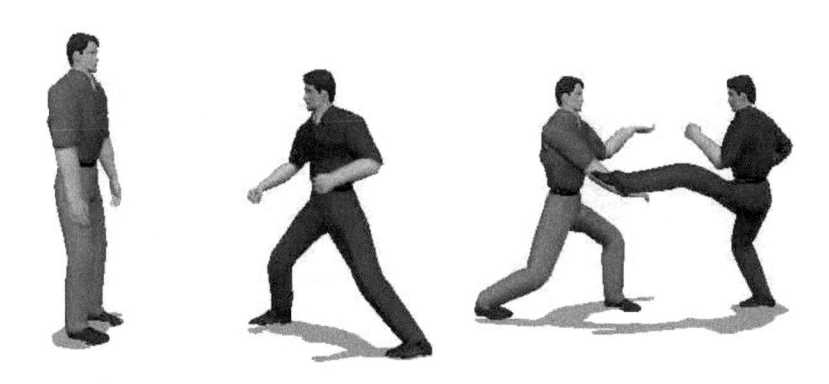

The Attacker prepares to punch.
Attacker executes a left front snap kick. The Defender steps back with the right foot into a front stance as he executes a left palm up block and a right palm down block.

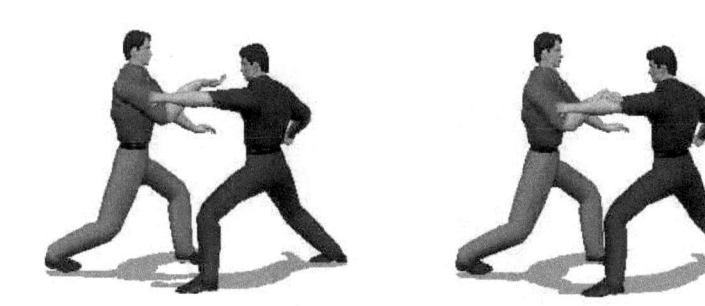

The Attacker sets forward with the left foot into a front stance as he executes a left punch. The Defender executes left palm down block and a right palm up block.
The Defender hooks his right hand over the Attacker's left arm.

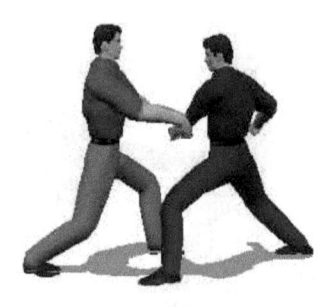

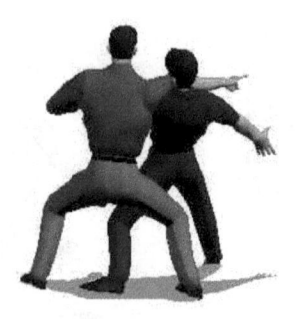

The Defender starts to circle the Attacker's left arm down and across.

The Defender steps behind the Attacker in a horse stance as he transfers the Attacker's left arm to his right and holds it with a hook. Extending the right arm across the Attacker's neck the Defender 'splits' the Attacker.

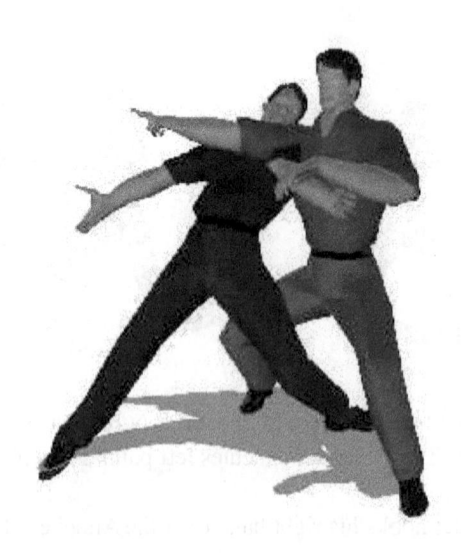

Here is a different viewpoint of the last move.

APPLICATION NUMBER THIRTY-FIVE

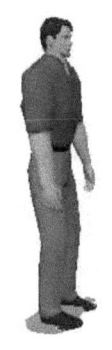

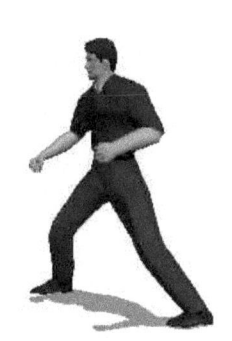

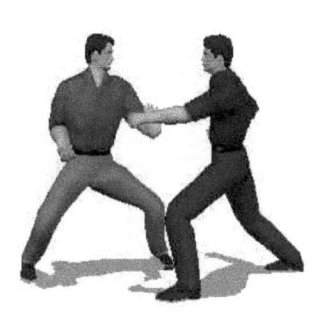

The Attacker prepares to punch.

The Attacker steps forward with the left foot into a front stance as he executes a left punch. The Defender steps back with the right foot into a horse stance as he executes a left palm block.

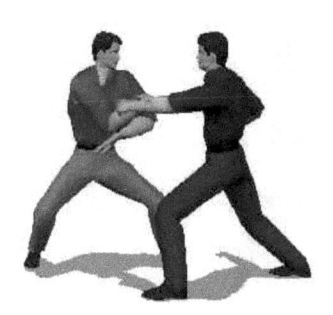

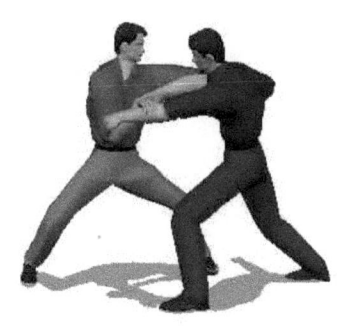

    The Defender reaches under his arm and grabs the Attacker's wrist. The Defender's left arm prepares for an elbow spike.
    The Defender pulls the Attacker's left arm with his right hand as he executes a left elbow strike.

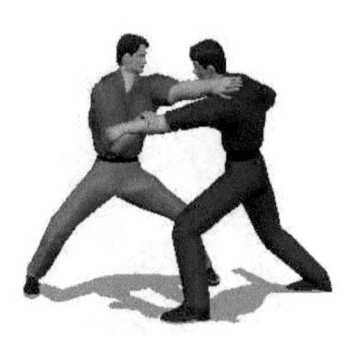

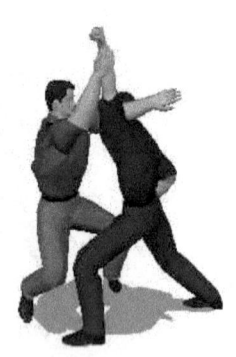

The Defender Defender straightens out his left arm on the side of the Attacker's neck and prepares to push the Attacker's left arm up and around.

The Defender moves forward with the right foot as he pushes down on the Attacker's neck with his left arm and up and back on the Attacker's left arm with his right arm. It is very important that you do not push down on the Attacker's arm, that would leave him enough wiggle room to let him escape. The Defender will seek a wrist lock as he comes around (see next illustration.)

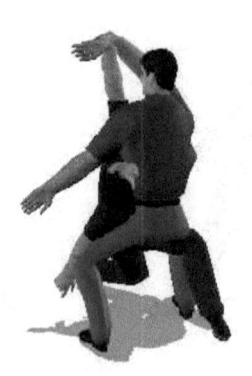

The Defender completes moving around the Attacker with his right leg into a horse stance. The Attacker should be severely crumpled and bent, as you can see from the illustration. We're talking potential broken neck, severely cranked spine, left shoulder out of socket, knee smashed into the ground, and complete and utter control out of the Attacker. The secret to this technique is to achieve total vertical with the Attacker's left arm and drive it downward. I love this technique.

APPLICATION NUMBER THIRTY-SIX

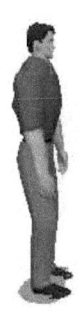

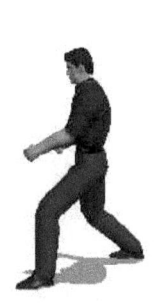

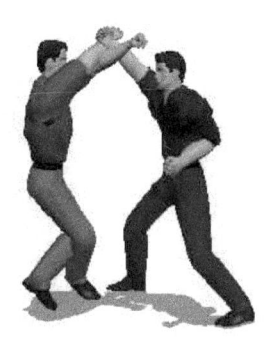

The Attacker prepares to attack (as if with a club).

The Attacker steps forward with the right foot into a front stance as he executes an overhead clubbing attack. The Defender steps in front of his left foot with his right foot into an x-stance as he executes a high crossed wrist block. (SPECIAL NOTE: In the beginning, make contact, but, as you get better, don't block, just look like you're going to, then absorb the Attacker's motion by going with it. This is a little bit Aikido, but okay considering that advanced students should be not only looking at other arts, but absorbing them constantly).

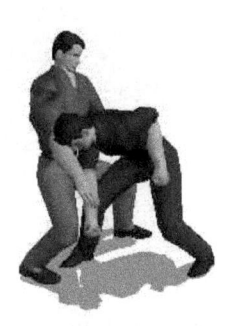

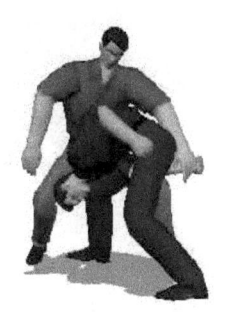

The Defender keeps moving to the left by stepping with his left foot into a horse stance as he pushes the Attacker's club arm down with his right arm.

The Defender pushes the Attacker's arm between his legs and catches it with his left hand. If you can't figure out what to do now you're an idiot.

If you can't push the hand through the Attacker should be bent over, and it is a wonderful time to just hammer the heck out of his back.

APPLICATION NUMBER THIRTY-SEVEN

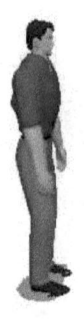

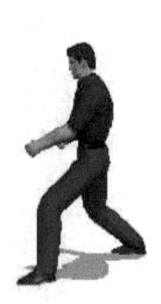

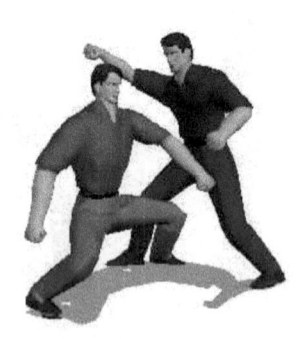

The Attacker prepares to punch to the face.

The Attacker steps forward with the right foot into a front stance as he executes a punch to the face. The Defender steps forward and *under the punch* into a horse stance as he executes double low blocks. Done in this fashion the block becomes a hammer, and the left one sort of happens to strike the Attacker in the groin. This technique requires split second timing. Too fast and the Attacker will hold back. Too slow and you'll take one to the face.

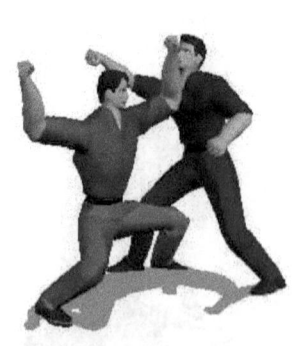

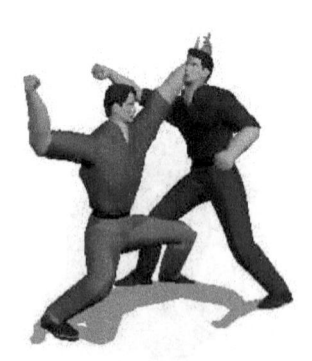

The Defender executes a double shoulder high outward block. Done in this fashion, the blocks become backfists, and the left one just happens to strike the Attacker in the face.

The Defender straightens his left arm on the side of the Attacker's neck.

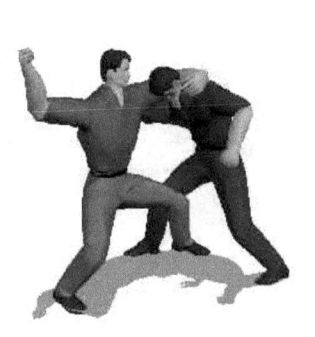

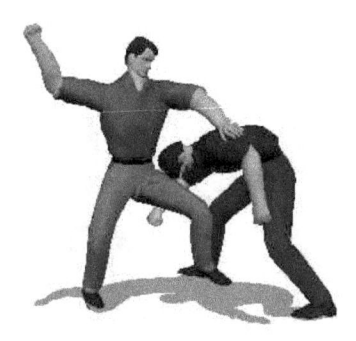

The Defender hooks the left arm around the Attacker's head and begins to pull. The Defender may start straightening up so as to put body weight behind the pull.

The Defender has succeeded in bending the Attacker over. He prepares to execute a hammerfist to the Attacker's back.

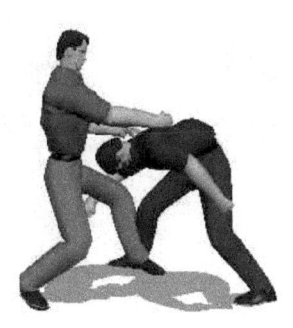

The Defender executes a hammerfist to the Attacker's back. One should study the anatomy of the spine so as to best create effect on the Attacker's structure.

Now, what if The Attacker resists the pull to his head? What would you do? Solving this you should examine every technique you have and figure in one factor: at what point can the Attacker go in a direction that is opposite to what is planned for him? This can happen at one place, many places, or no places. Past this you should figure out angles of resistance that are not opposite, but other than the planned or opposite direction.

APPLICATION NUMBER THIRTY-EIGHT

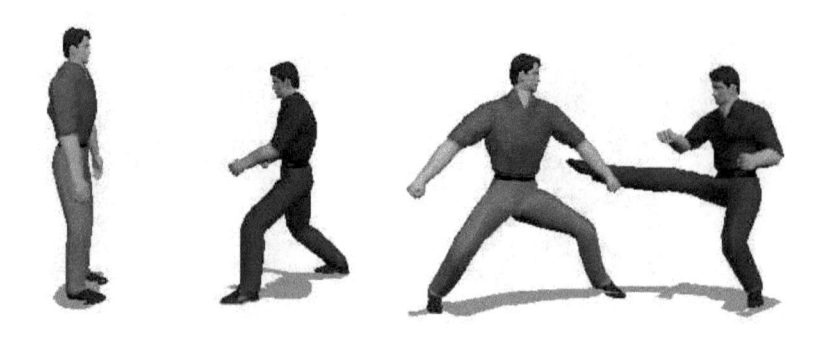

The Attacker prepares to kick.

The Attacker executes a right snap kick. The Defender steps back with the right foot into a horse stance as he executes double low blocks.

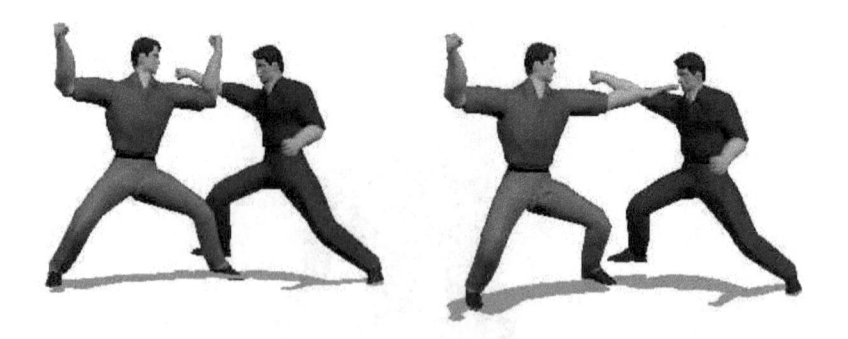

The Attacker sets forward with the right foot into a front stance as he executes a right punch to the face. The Defender executes double shoulder high outward blocks.

The Defender extends his left arm.

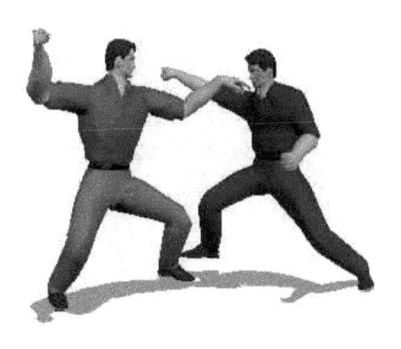

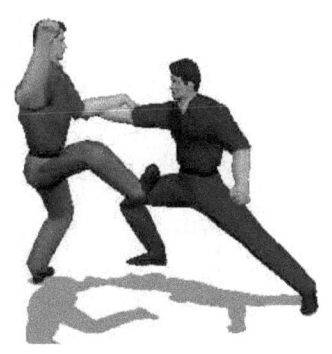

The Defender hooks the Attacker's right arm with his left hand.

The Defender pulls the Attacker's right arm as he executes a right foot stomp to the Attacker's right knee. (What would happen if the Defender simply swept the Attacker?) Is that a better technique? Or worse? What would determine which technique should be chosen?)

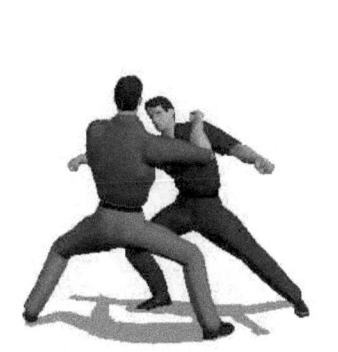

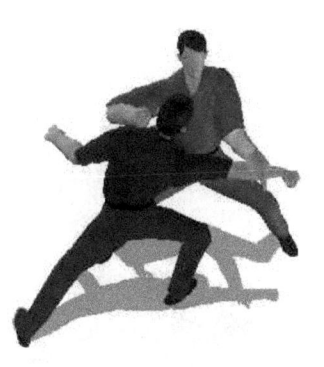

The Defender sets forward with the right foot into a horse stance as he pulls on the attacker's arm and executes a right hammer to the Attacker's left collar bone. (The collar bone is only as thick as a couple of pencils. It is free floating, but it should be simple to break, which would take that side of the Attacker out of the action.)

View of the last position from the other side.

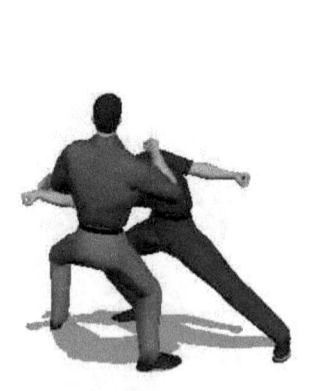

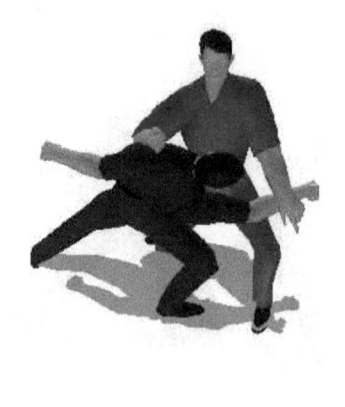

The Defender continues to pull the Attacker's right arm and pushes with his right arm. The Attacker, who should be shocked by a kicked knee and a broken collar bone, is pulled forward and twisted.
View of the last position from the other side.

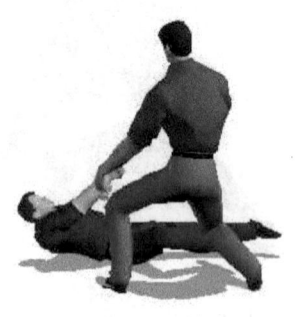

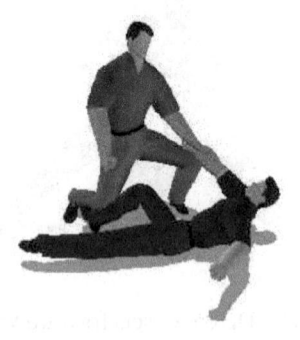

The Attacker is flung to the ground on his back.
View of the last position from the other side.

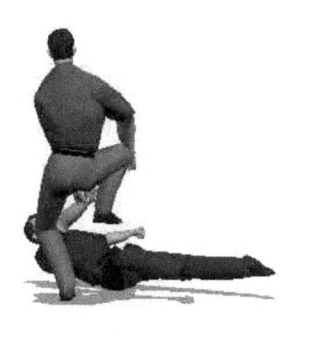

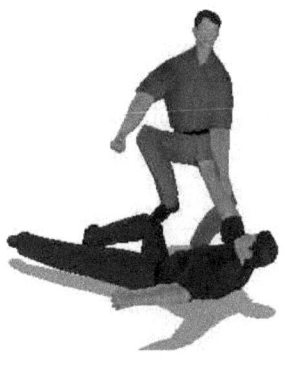

The Defender raises his right foot.
View of the last position from the other side.

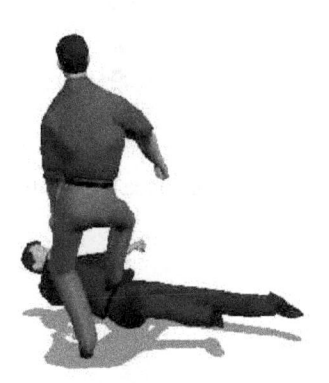

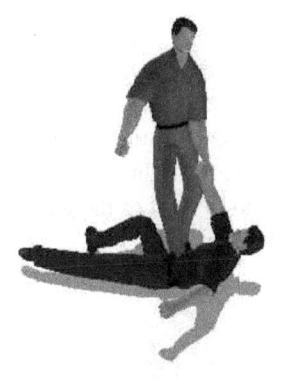

The Defender executes a particular brutal stomp. The crowd cheers.
View of the last position from the other side.

This application has roots in jujitsu. It would probably be more karate to simply slap the Attacker on the ear after breaking his collar bone. This would rupture his eardrum and thoroughly discombobulate his semi circular canals (balance), but aside from looking at all artistic potentials in the matter, consider that you might not want to damage the fellow. What if he is just your drunk brother-in-law? This is a matter of ethics and responsibility, and I guarantee that you won't reach the higher levels of the art unless you root yourself in ethics and responsibility.

NOHAI

Nohai (sometimes called Rohai) means 'Vision of a White Crane.' It is marked by a series of steps and jumps to a crane stance. Imagine having to leap from rock to slippery rock in the middle of a stream and you will understand the purpose. You will gain balance and grace. More importantly, you will learn to 'peg' your ground suddenly and surely.

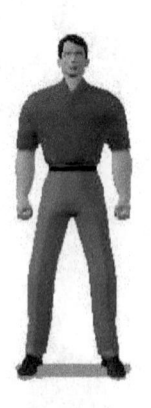

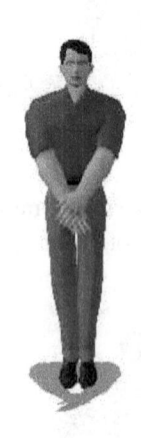

Stand in a natural stance.
Bring the right foot next to the left foot as you place the left hand over the right hand in front of the groin.

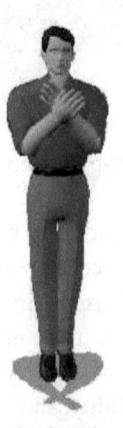

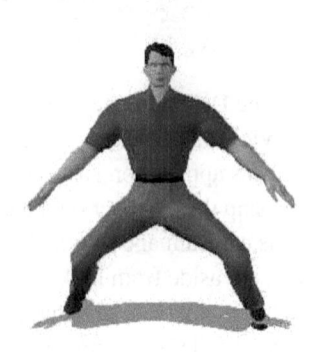

Bring the hands up.
Step to the right with the right foot into a horse stance as you execute double low blocks to the sides. Make sure you breathe out when you expand, and in when you contract. Breath to the Tan Tien ('The One Point,' located approximately two inches below the navel).

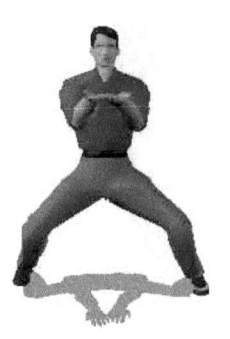

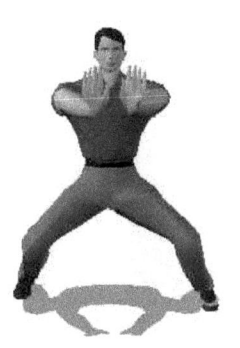

Bring the hands up, the palms should be horizontal. Breath in. Breath out as you push forward. There should be much dynamic tension, as if you are pushing a car.

There won't be a lot of applications for this form, but as you have seen, there is much practice of breathing, tension, relaxation, balance, and so on, in this form.

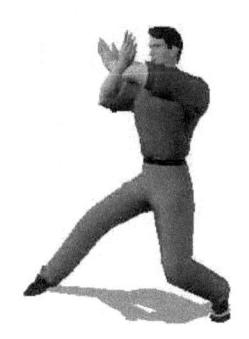

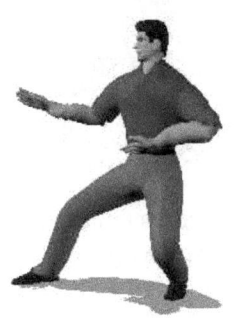

Bring the right foot in as you pivot towards a back stance facing to the right. The left hand protects the face as the right hand prepares for a knife block.

Assume a back stance as you execute a right knife block.

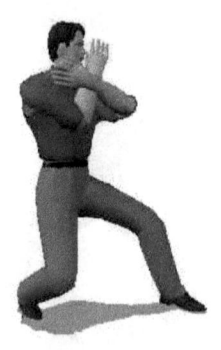

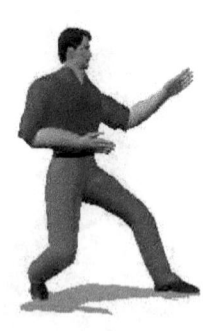

Pivot to the left, the right hand protects the face as the left hand prepares for a knife block.

Assume a back stance as you execute a left knife block.

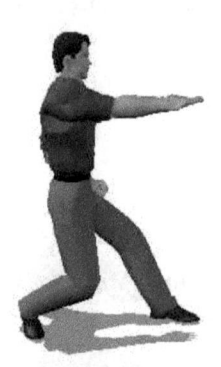

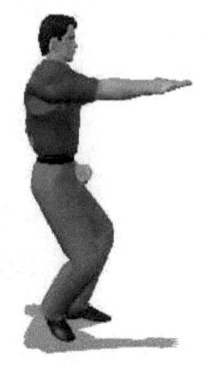

Execute a right spear hand.
Bring the right foot up next to the left foot.

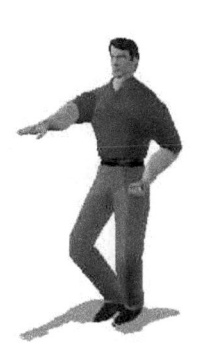

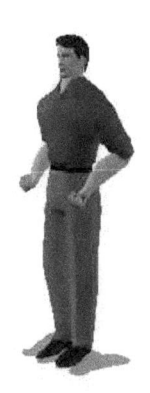

Turn 135 degrees to the right. The hand should be out during the turn, and the whole body should turn as one unit. The knees are still bent.

Straighten up as you retract your right hand.

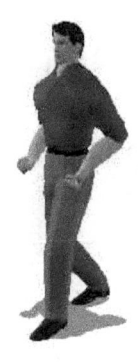

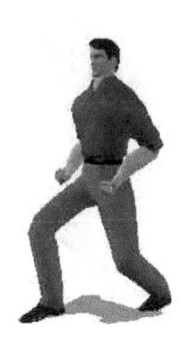

Take a left step.
Take a right step.

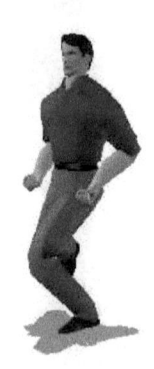

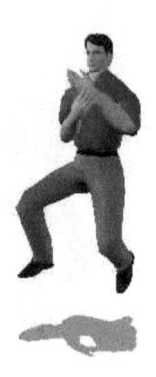

Hook the left foot behind the left knee in a crane stance. Leap backwards. The hands should prepare for crane positioning.

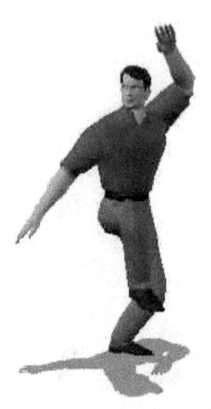

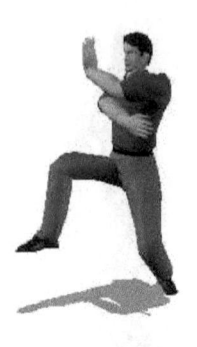

Land on the left leg, the right leg raised to the side, the right arm in a low knife block, the left hand in a high knife block.

Move forward, the left hand covering the face, the right hand preparing for a chop.

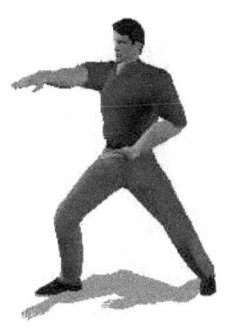

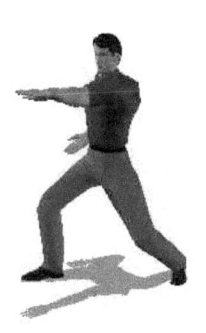

Land in a front stance as you execute a right chop.
Execute a left spear.

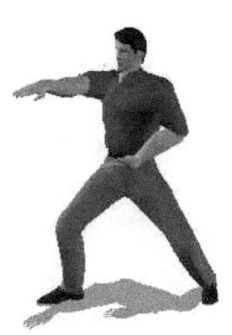

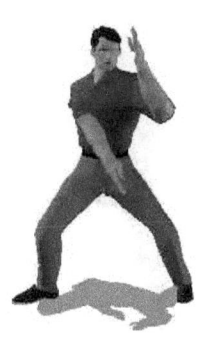

Execute a right spear.
The right hand circles down and the left hand circles up.

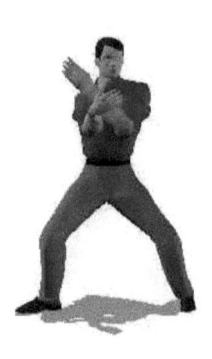

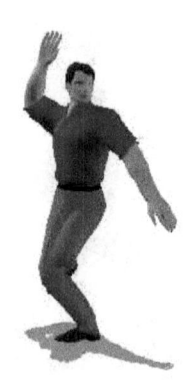

The hands continue to circle.
Hook the left foot behind the right knee as you execute a left low knife block and a right high knife block.

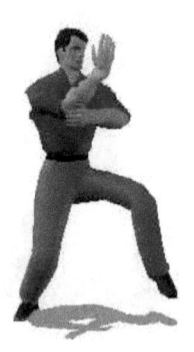

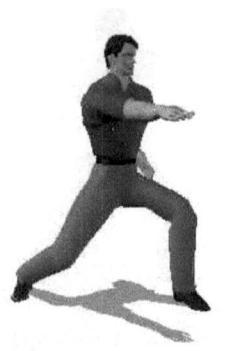

Fall to the right, the right hand protects the face and the left hand prepares to chop.
Execute a right spear.

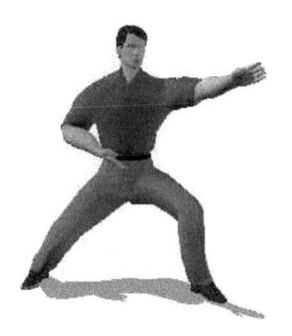

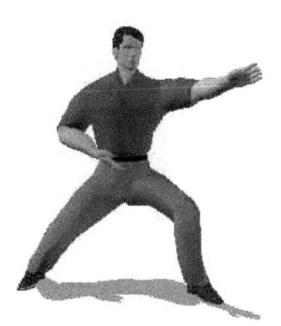

Execute a left spear.
Land in a front stance as you execute a left chop.

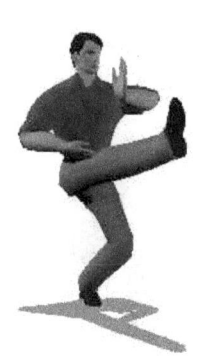

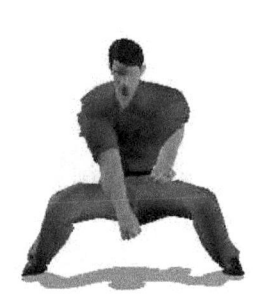

Cover the face with a left palm block as you execute a right leg raise.
Bring the leg back to a position so you are in a horse stance facing squarely to the front. Simultaneously, execute a right punch towards the floor. Some people like to punch all the way to the floor. Just don't slaughter your horse stance when you do this.

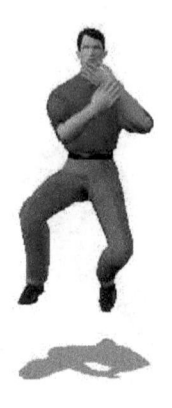

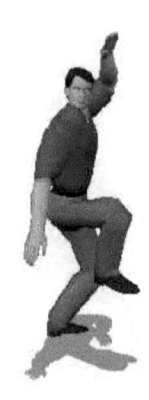

Leap up and backward as you prepare the hands for a crane position.

Land on the left leg in a crane stance as you execute a right low knife block and a left high knife block. The right knee should be raised to the left.

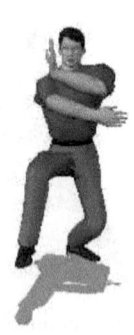

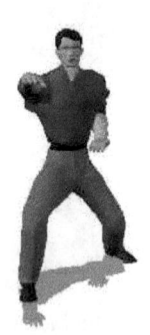

Fall forward as you protect the face with your left hand and prepare the right hand for a chop.

Land in a front stance as you execute a right chop.

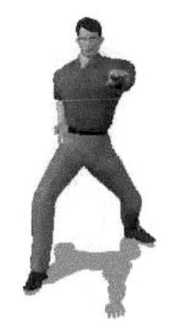

Execute a left spear.
Execute a right spear.

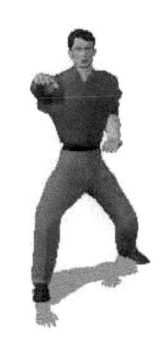

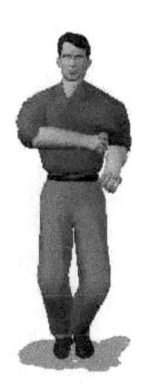

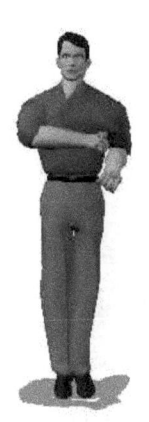

Bring the right foot back to the next as you bring the right hand back and across the body. The knees should be bent.
Straighten up.

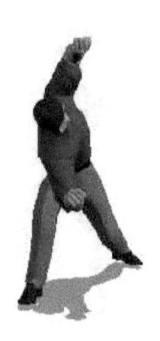

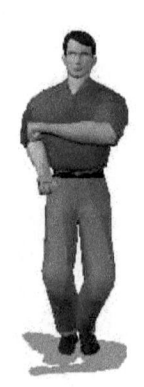

Step forward with the right foot into a front stance as you execute a left over punch and right under punch.

Bring the right foot back next to the left foot as you retract the right hand to the hip and the left hand across the body. The knees should be bent.

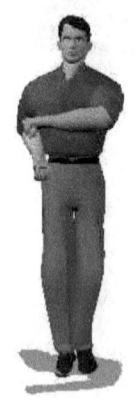

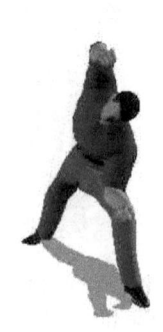

Straighten up.

Step forward with the left foot into a front stance as you execute a right punch over and a left punch under.

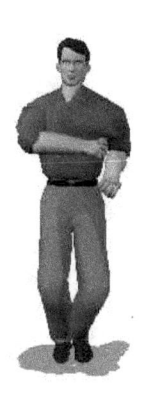

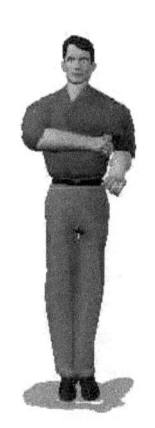

Bring the left foot back next to the right foot as you retract the left hand to the hip and position the left hand across the body. The knees should be bent.
Straighten up.

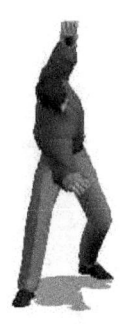

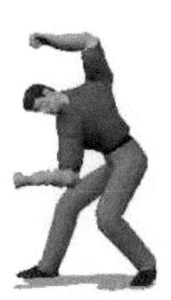

Step forward with the right foot into a *back stance* as you execute a right punch over and a left punch under.
Side view of the last position.

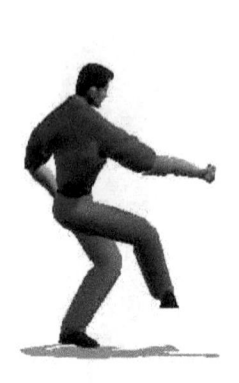

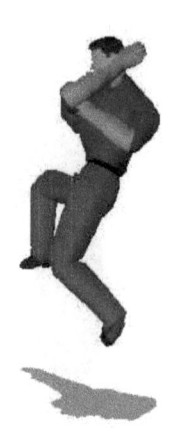

Swing the right foot and the right hand down and towards the rear. This is necessary to enable the body to achieve the coming jump spin.

Jump high and to the rear. As you spin prepare the right hand for a knife block.

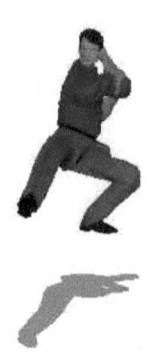

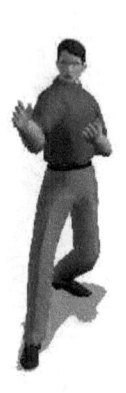

Almost ready to land.

The key here is to get enough lift by swinging your leg upwards in the first place.

Land in a back stance as you execute a right knife block.

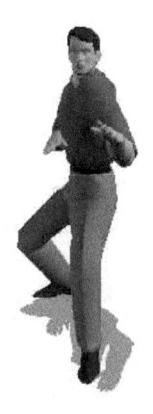

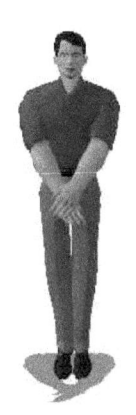

Step back with the right foot into a back stance as you execute a left knife block.

Return to the beginning position.

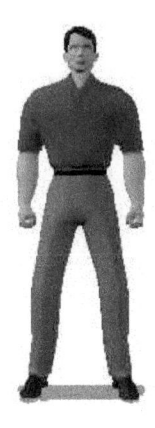

Return to the natural position.

NUMBER THIRTY-NINE

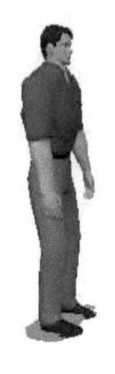

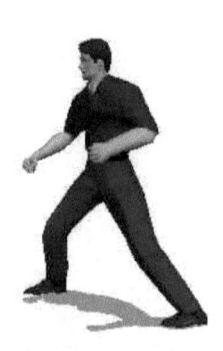

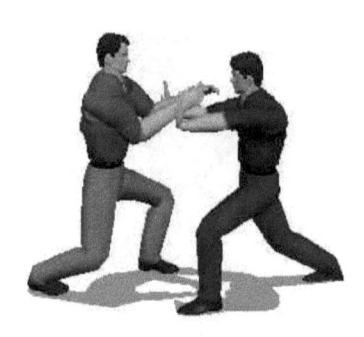

The Attacker prepares to push.

The Attacker steps forward with the left foot into a front stance as he executes a two handed push to the shoulders. The Defender starts to step back with the right foot as he raises both hands between the Attacker's arms.

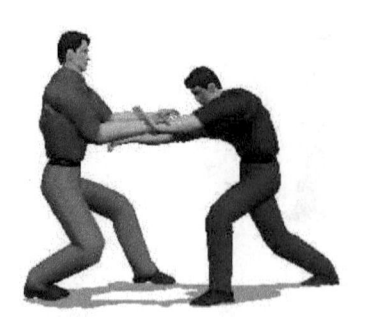

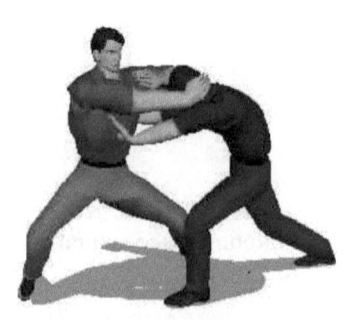

The Defender assumes a back stance as he pulls both of the Attacker's arms down. The Defender must be careful not to get himself headbutted.

The Defender pivots into a horse stance as he places his right hand on the side of the Attacker's head and executes a left elbow strike to the side of the Attacker's head.

APPLICATION NUMBER FORTY

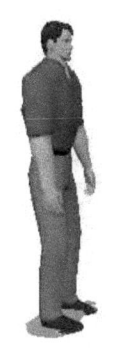

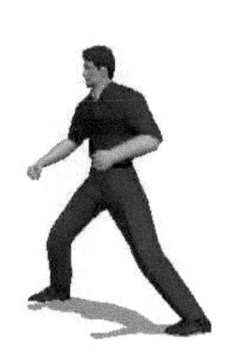

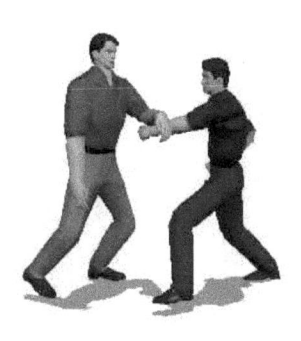

The Attacker prepares to punch.

The Attacker steps forward with the left foot into a front stance as he executes a left punch. The Defender steps backward with the right foot as he circles the left hand over the Attacker's arm.

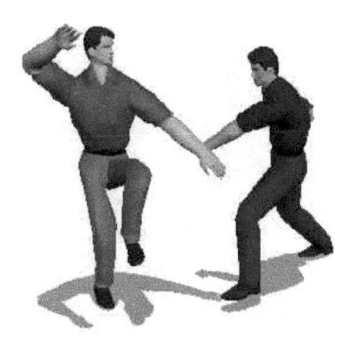

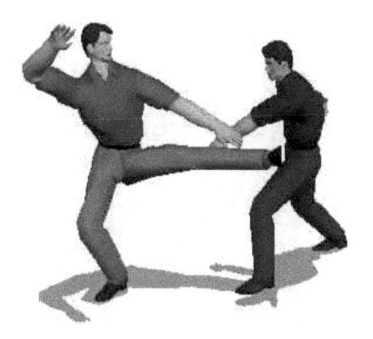

The Defender assumes a crane stance as he pushes the Attacker's arm down and to the side.

The Defender executes a left side thrust kick.

Knowing how to control distance is crucial to being effective in the martial arts. If a fellow is a better kicker, close to punching, throwing, etc. If he is better at punching, as one would assume from the above technique, the Defender must increase the distance. This is sometimes difficult because rule number one, when a fight starts, is that distance will collapse. But being of sufficient presence of mind to undo rule number one means that one is attaining the true calm of mind necessary to great martial artists.

APPLICATION NUMBER FORTY-ONE

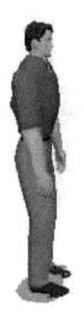

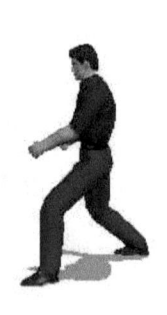

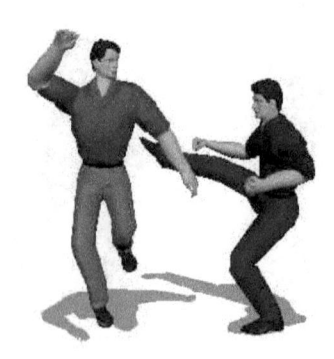

The Attacker prepares to kick

The Attacker executes a right front snap kick. The Defender assumes a crane stance as he executes a right high knife block and a left low knife block.

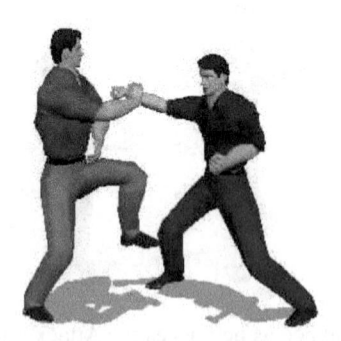

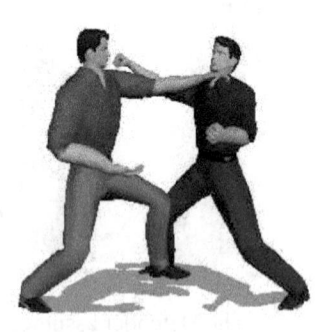

The Attacker sets down in a front stance as he executes a right punch. The Defender moves into the Attacker as he executes a right palm block.

The Defender sets into a front stance with the right foot forward as he executes a left chop to the neck. The collar bone may be a better target. Also, it's good to take out his knee with your own knee.

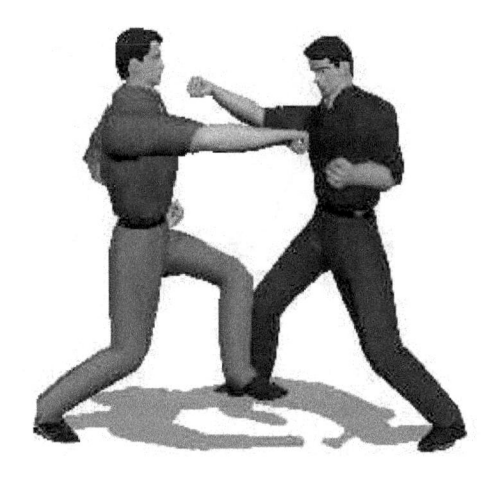

The Defender executes a right punch.

This technique teaches one the concept of 'split' timing. If you can 'split' time a technique you are starting to perceive the techniques in 'now' time, which is a very good thing.

APPLICATION NUMBER FORTY-TWO

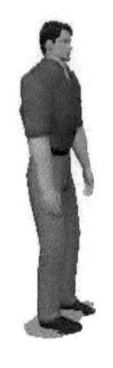

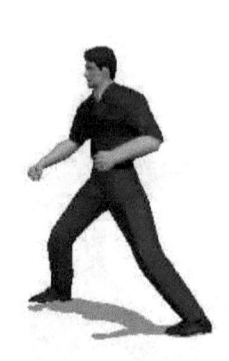

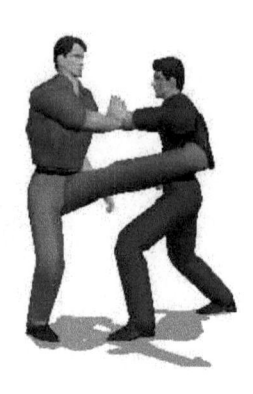

The Attacker prepares to punch.

The Attacker steps forward with the left foot into a front stance as he executes a left punch. The Defender executes a right cross palm block and a left leg raise.

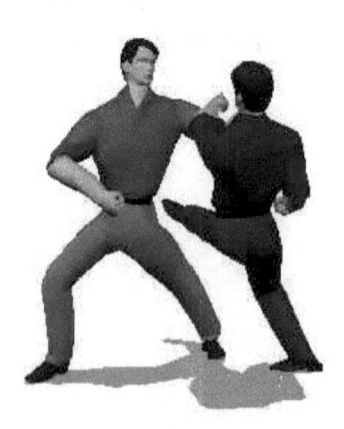

The Defender thrusts the left foot back through the Attacker's left leg into a front stance. At the same time he executes a left palm to the Attacker's chest.

This is a very aggressive technique. To protect your partner you may grab his left biceps with your right hand and make sure he doesn't hit the ground too hard. As he learns how to fall, you can ease off letting him down easy.

BOTSAI

Botsai means 'Defending the Fortress.' It is a very strong form, and you should see internal energy manifesting as you practice it.

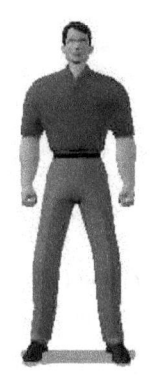

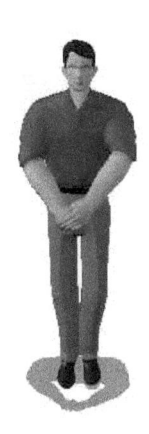

Begin in a natural stance.
Bring the right foot next to the left as you cover the right fist with the left hand in front of the groin.

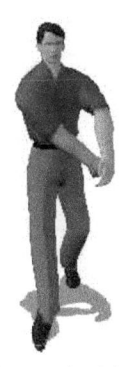

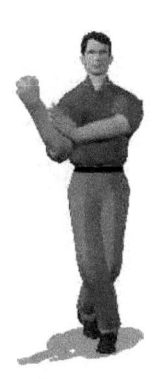

Step forward with the right foot as you move the arms to the left in preparation.
Stomp lightly on the right foot as you bring the left foot up behind it in an x-stance. Simultaneously execute a right augmented outward middle block.

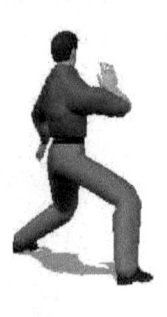

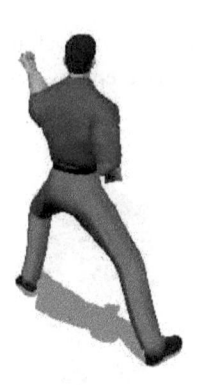

Step back and to the right with the left foot. The left arm should move as a sweeping parry (dangling forearm) to cover the groin and the right palm should cover the face. You shouldn't look before you move because this will destroy your CBM (see article on Coordinated Body Motion to Find the True Art); rather, you should move the body as one unit, which will create internal energy.

Finish the move into a front stance as you execute a left middle outward block.

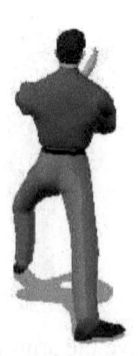

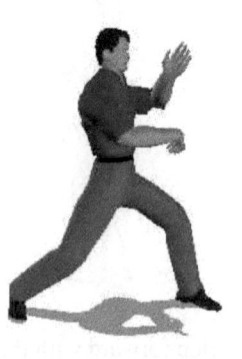

Open the left palm to cover the face (very quick and subtle, most people won't see it) as you twist the body to the left. The right hand should be preparing for an outward block by traveling through a parry (dangling forearm).

Side view of last position.

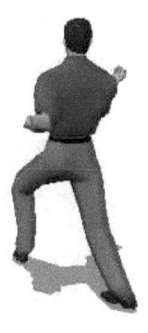

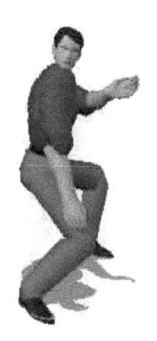

Complete the twist (keeping the weight firmly on the left foot as you execute a right outward middle block.

Step to left (behind your body) with the right foot. This will set up a front stance to the front. Simultaneously swing the the right arm down to cover the groin and move the left hand into a palm block to cover the face.

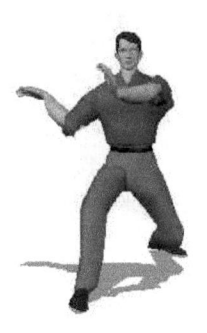

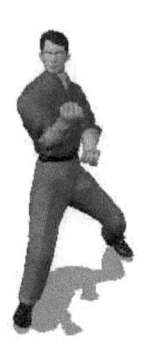

Complete the turn into a front stance. The left hand executes the palm block and the right hand prepares for an inward middle block.

Execute a right inward middle block.

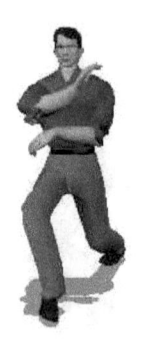

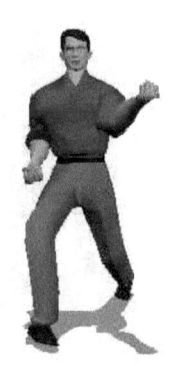

Twist to the right as you open the right hand into a quick palm to cover the face. The left hand should be moving through a dangling forearm block.

Complete the twist as you execute a left outward middle block. You should be pointing the rear foot at the front foot when you do these twisting stances. It is okay to drag the rear foot slightly forward, but don't let the body rise up. The point here is to put the hip into the block.

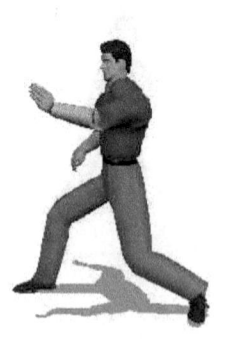

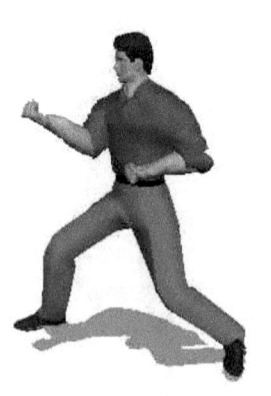

Step to the right. The arms should travel through a left palm block and a right dangling forearm.

Assume a front stance. The right arm should circle out, up and in to execute a right inward middle block.

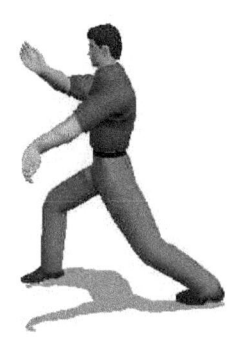

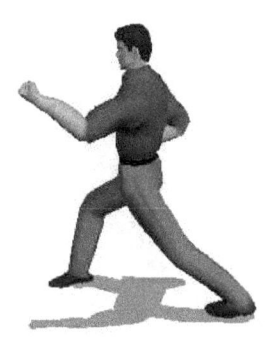

Twist to the right as you open the right palm and execute a left dangling forearm.

Complete the twist as you execute a left outward middle block.

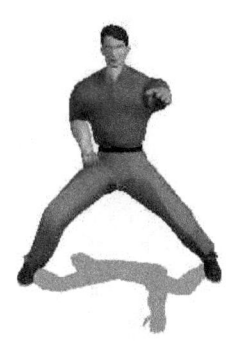

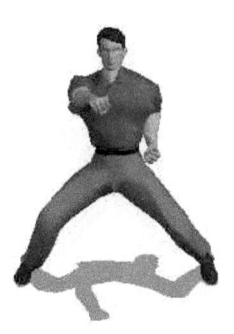

'Stump' the right foot to the left (aligning a horse stance to the front) as you execute a left chop. Stumping means that you don't shift the weight, but rather lift the foot and replace it before you can fall.

Execute a right punch.

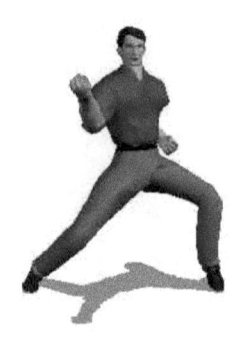

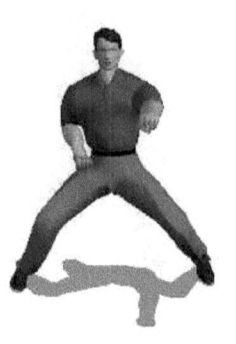

Twist to the left into a front stance as you execute a left outward middle block.

Snap the hips to the right as you execute a left punch.

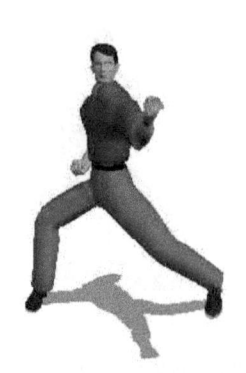

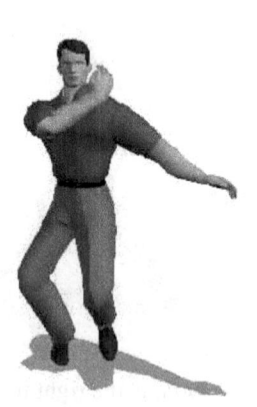

Twist to the right into a front stance as you execute a right outward middle block.

Bring the left foot up as you raise the right hand to cup the ear and extend the left hand low and to the side. These movements prepare for a knife block.

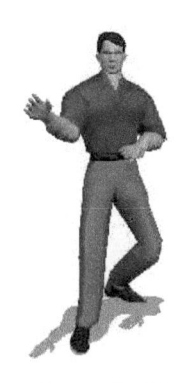

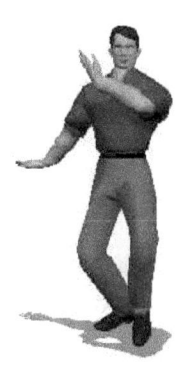

Step forward with the right foot into a back stance as you execute a right knife block.

Move the left foot forward into a cat stance as you raise the left hand to cup the ear and extend the right hand down and to the side.

Every movement should set up a twist to add power to the next movement.

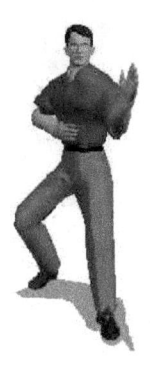

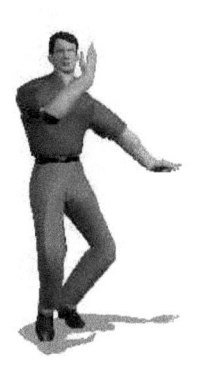

Continue stepping forward with the left foot into a back stance as you execute a left knife block.

Move the right foot forward to a cat stance as you raise the left hand and extend the right hand.

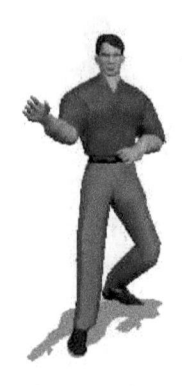

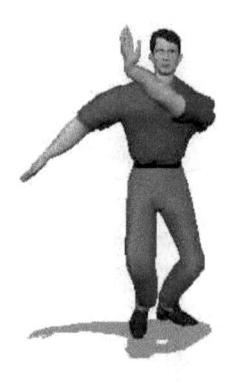

Continue moving the right foot forward into a back stance as you execute a right knife block.

Step back with the right foot into a cat stance as you raise the left hand and extend the right hand.

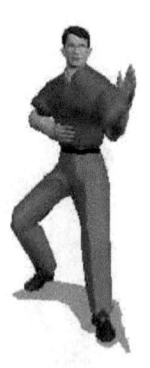

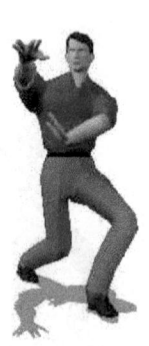

Finish stepping back into a back stance as you execute a left knife block.

Shift forward onto the left foot as you twist to the right. At the same time, execute a left low palm block and a right spear. The right spear should have a split between the middle and ring (fourth) fingers.

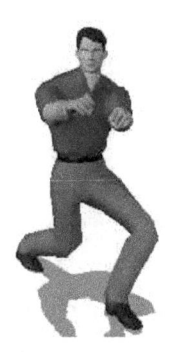

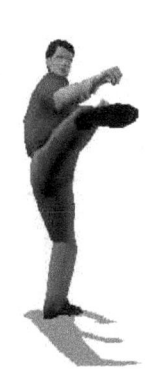

Close the fists as if reaching and grabbing.
Execute a right side thrust kick to the front.

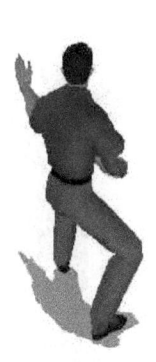

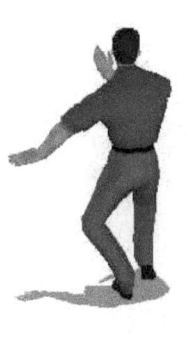

Retract the right foot and stomp it exactly where the left foot was standing. The left foot shoots to the rear as you assume a back stance. Bring the hands *over* and down into a knife block.

Step forward with the right foot into a cat stance as you raise the right hand and extend the left hand.

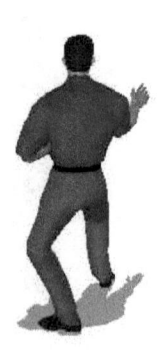

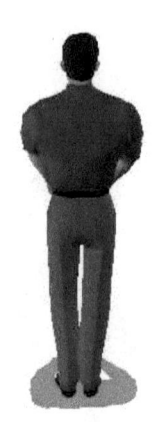

Continue stepping forward with the right foot into a back stance as you execute a right knife block.

Bring the right foot back next to the left foot. At the same time bring the fists in front of the thighs.

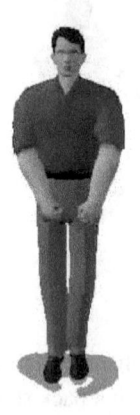

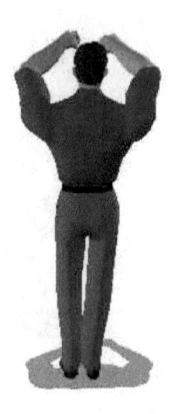

View of last position from the opposite side.
Execute double high blocks.

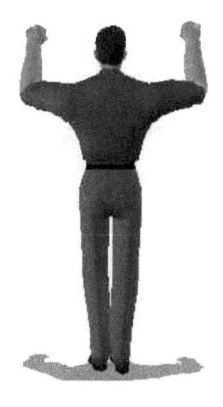

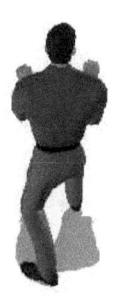

Execute double shoulder high inverted outward blocks.

Step forward with the right foot as you bring the hands all the way around and into uppercuts to the midsection.

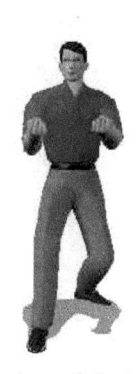

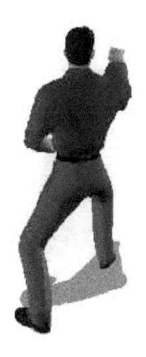

Rear view of the last position.

Step forward with the right foot into a front stance as you execute a right punch.

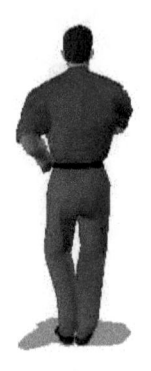

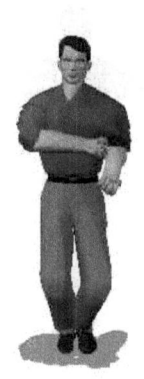

Place the right foot next to the left foot as you move the right arm parallel across the front of the body.

Rear view of the last position.

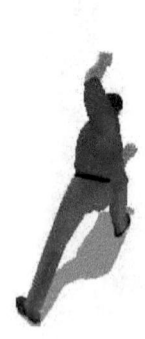

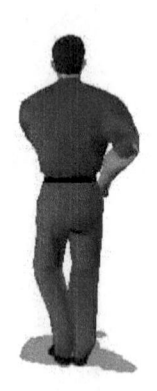

Step forward with the right foot into a front stance as you execute a right under punch and a left over punch.

Place the right foot next to the left foot as you move the right fist to the hip and the left arm parallel across the body.

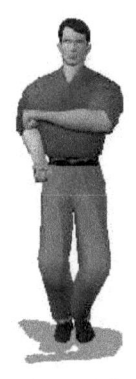

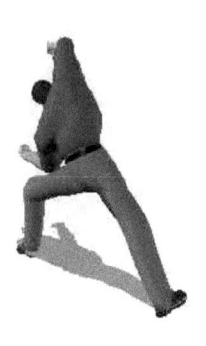

Rear view of the last position.

Step forward with the left foot into a front stance as you execute a left under punch and a right over punch.

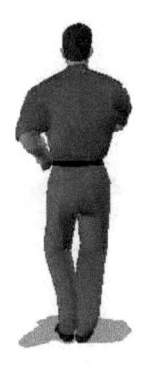

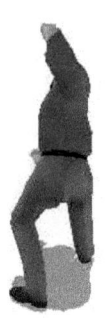

Place the left foot next to the right foot as you retract the left fist to the hip and move the right arm parallel across the body.

Move the right foot forward into a *back stance* as you execute a right under punch and a left over punch.

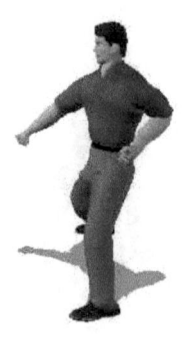

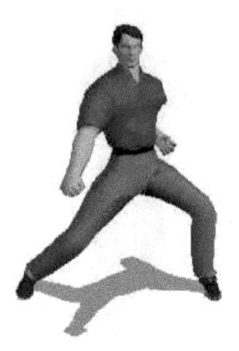

Stump the left foot back slightly so it is in line with the right foot. Twist to the left through a front stance as you execute an inverted low block. *This movement is done slow and with much tension and with complete concentration on CBM (the whole body as one unit.)*

Side view of the last position. Remember, there is no focus, this is a transition posture.

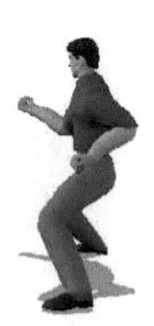

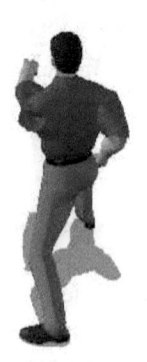

Continue with the slow tension by twisting back to the right into a horse stance as you execute a right middle outward block.

Stump the right foot slightly to the right (not a full two track, shoulder width stance, more of a single track line up) into a front stance as you execute a left punch.

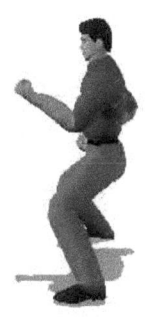

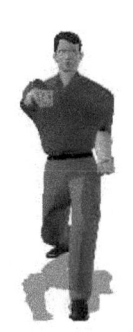

Move the left foot back slightly into an in line horse stance as you execute a left middle outward block. *Do this with slow CBM.*

Stump the left foot slightly to the rear, creating a single track front stance, as you execute a right punch.

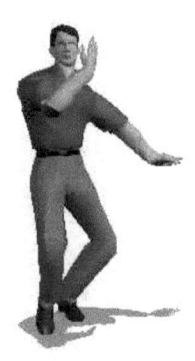

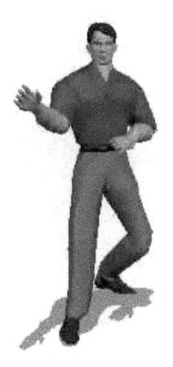

Step forward with the right foot into a cat stance as you raise the right hand and extend the left hand.

Continue stepping with the right foot into a back stance as you execute a right knife block.

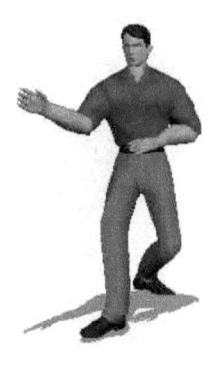

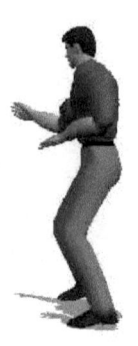

Slowly, with intention to CBM, turn the right foot to the right (forty-five degrees outward). Turn the right knife hand in perfect time with the foot.

Step forward with the left foot into an hourglass stance. The knife hand should be totally one with the body. Not a lot of tension is required, just attention to detail.

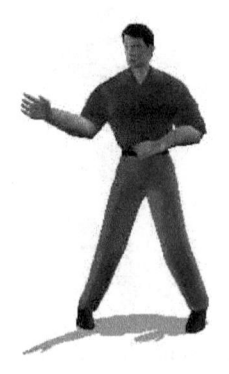

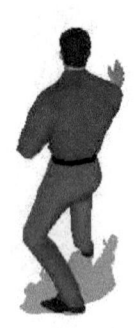

Side view of the last position.

Turn the right foot to the right and shift into a back stance. Again, the knife hand and the foot point the intention to CBM the movement.

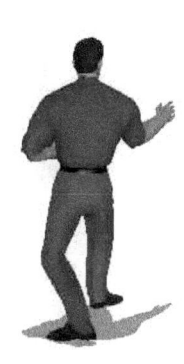

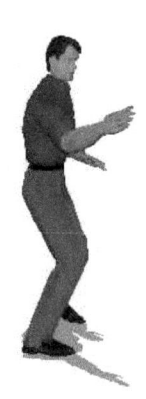

Turn the right foot and the right knife hand out 45 degrees. Step through with the left foot as you continue the CBMing.

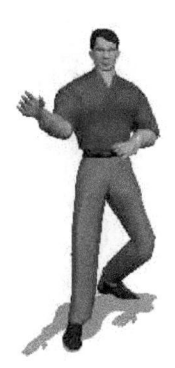

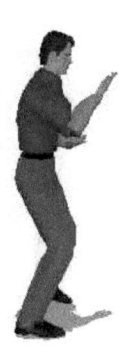

Pivot the right foot and shift into a back stance. The right knife hand stays pointed in the same direction as the right foot.

Pivot to the left into an hourglass stance. The right hand should move with the foot, but this time as an inward knife block.

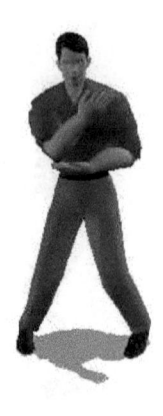

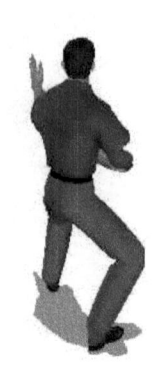

Side view of last position.
Continue to pivot into a back stance with a left knife block.

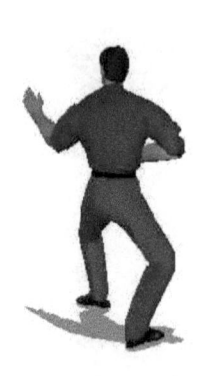

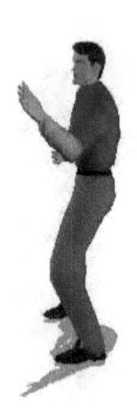

Turn the left foot outward and the left knife block.
Step forward with the right foot and pivot into an hourglass stance as you continue to move the right knife block.

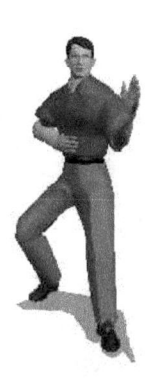

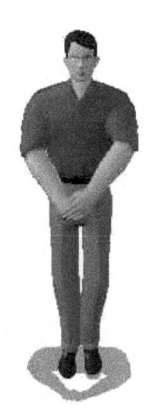

Pivot the left foot and shift into a back stance. The knife hand moves to the front.

Bring the right foot up next to the left foot and place the right fist under the cover of the left hand.

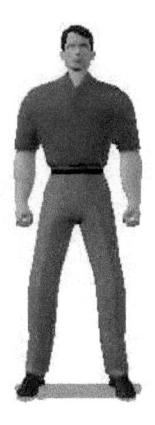

Step out to the right and relax the hands as you return to the starting position.

APPLICATION NUMBER FORTY-THREE

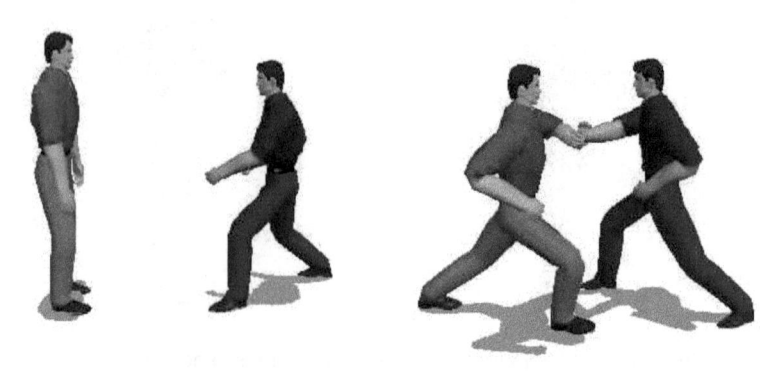

The Attacker prepares to punch.

The Attacker steps forward with the right foot as he executes a right punch. The Defender steps back with the left foot into a front stance as he executes a right cross palm block.

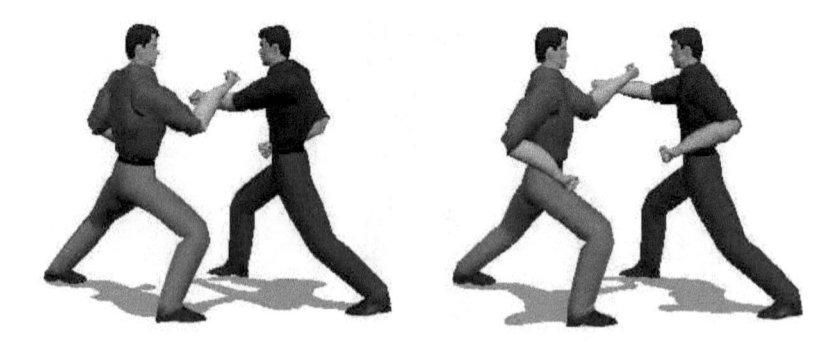

The Attacker executes a left punch. The Defender executes a right inward middle block.

The Attacker executes a right punch. The Defender executes a left middle outward block.

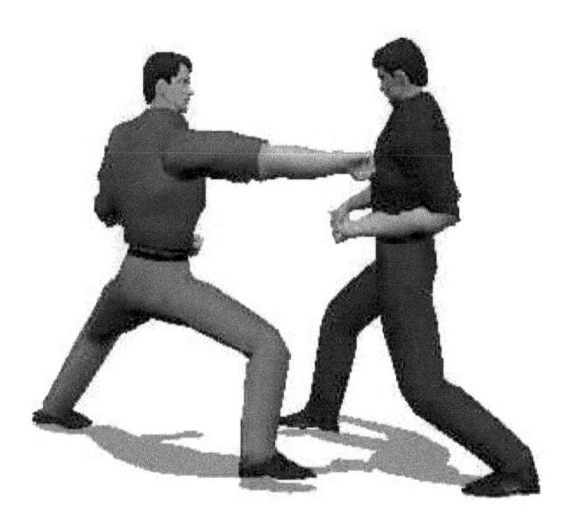

The Defender stumps the right foot slightly forward in a front stance as he executes a right punch.

This technique should be done faster and faster, until the student overcomes the idea that his blocks can't keep up. When the student gets the idea that his hands are moving independent of him, or that he is taking direct control of his hands, without the body, then he is doing this technique right.

APPLICATION NUMBER FORTY-FOUR

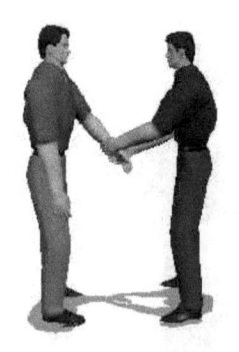

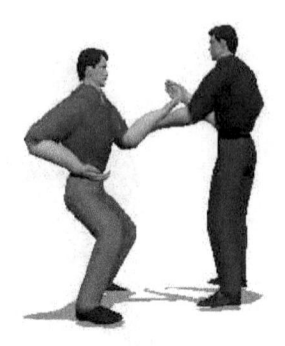

The Attacker executes a wrist grab with both hands.

The Defender steps to the right into a horse stance as he executes a left outward middle block.

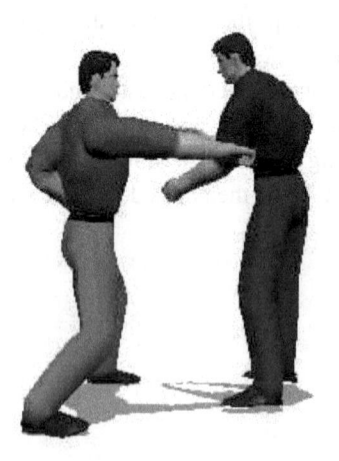

The Defender pivots to the left into a front stance as he executes a right punch.

Technically, one should never allow himself to be grabbed, one should move with the grab and thus avoid or counter it. However, this technique gives one confidence and strength in defeating any kind of wrist grab. The key is to change the angle of the grab. In this technique, for instance, the trick is to lower your hand and use the hips to twist up on the outside of the grab.

APPLICATION NUMBER FORTY-FIVE

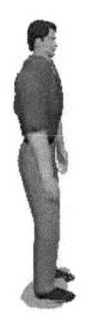

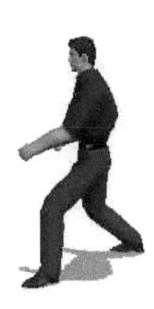

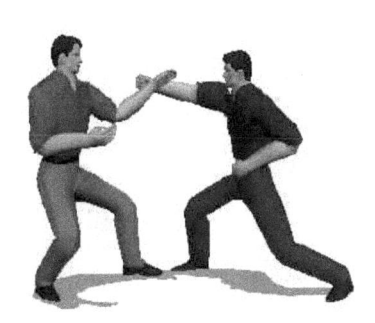

The Attacker prepares to strike.

The Attacker steps forward with the right foot into a front stance as he strikes with the right fist. The Defender steps back with the right foot into a back stance as he executes a left knife block.

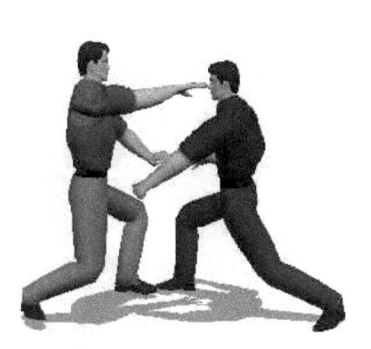

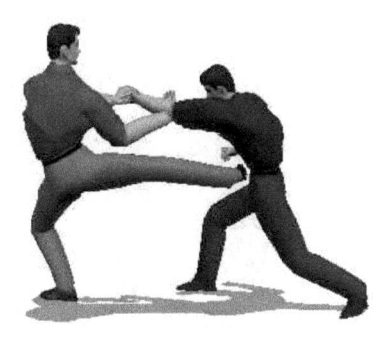

The Attacker executes a left punch. The Defender twists to the left into a front stance (more of a twisted kneeling stance) as he executes a left downward palm block and a right split finger spear to the eyes.

The Defender grabs the Attacker's arm and pulls as he executes a right side thrust kick to the midsection. You may have to pull the left foot back to give yourself room for this one. While this looks a bit awkward, remember that a good set up will hide your feet under his and your arms.

APPLICATION NUMBER FORTY-SIX

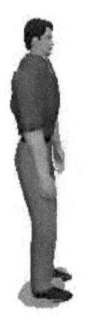

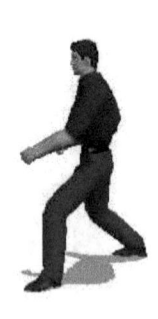

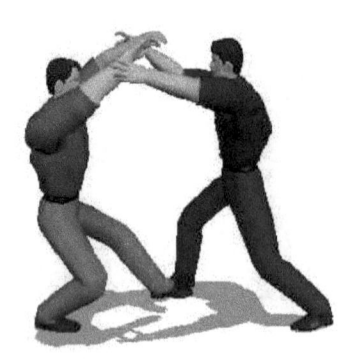

The Attacker prepares to execute a two hand grab for the neck.

The Attacker steps forward with the right foot into a front stance as he executes a two handed grab for the throat. The Defender steps back with the right foot into a back stance as he executes double high blocks.

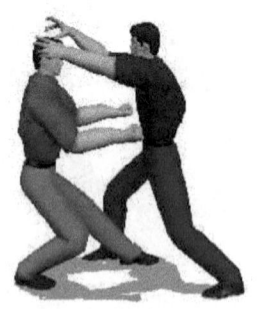

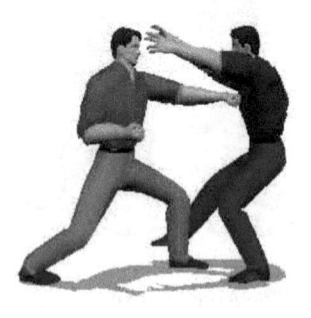

The Defender circles the arms around to execute a shuffling double uppercut to the midsection.

The Defender shifts into a front stance as he executes a left punch.

The idea here is that the arms must become very, very fast, and when the punch is your decided technique, you can move an Attacker back with authority.

APPLICATION NUMBER FORTY-SEVEN

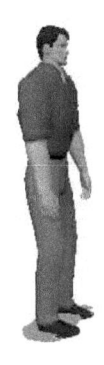

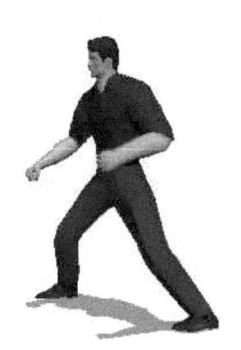

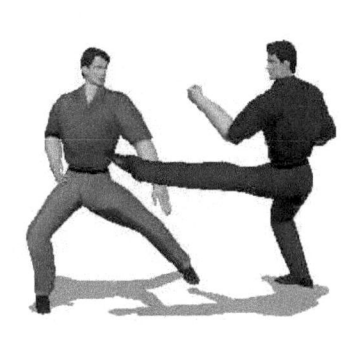

The Attacker prepares to kick.

The Attacker executes a left front snap kick. The Defender steps back and pivots to the right into a front stance as he executes a left inverted low block.

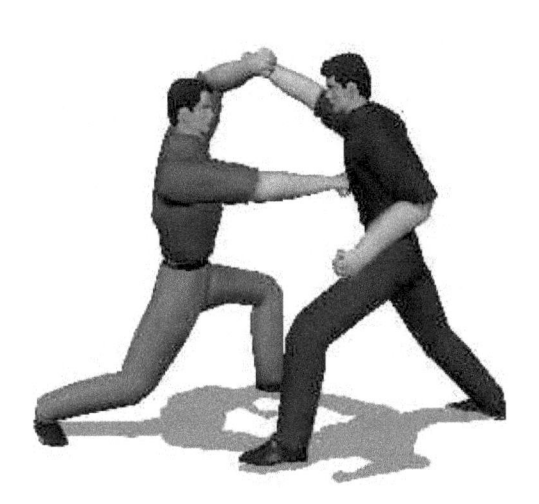

The Defender sets forward in a front stance as he executes a right punch to the face. The Defender pivots to the left into a front stance as he executes a left high block and a right punch.

Remember: it's not just the fist that snaps, and it's not just the hips. It's the whole body.

UMBE

Umbe means 'Darting Swallow.' As you do the form you can easily visualize a small bird arrowing through the air, darting under trees and over bushes.

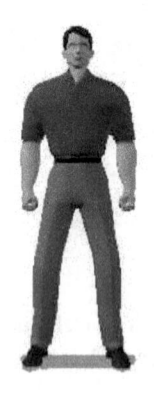

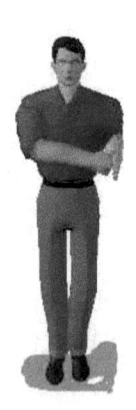

Stand in a natural stance.
Place the right foot next to the left foot. At the same time bring the right hand across the body and place the fist against the fingers.

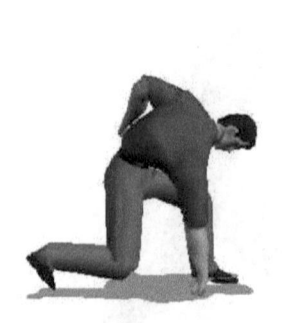

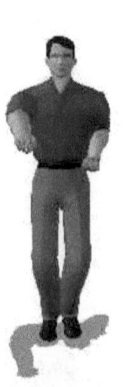

Step to the left with the left foot into a kneeling stance as you punch to within one inch of the ground. The right knee should also be within one inch of the ground.
Return the feet to the beginning position. The right arm should be outstretched and the body should be as one unit as you move to this position. The left hand should be cocked to the hip. the knees should remain bent.

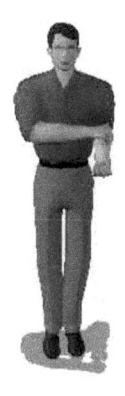

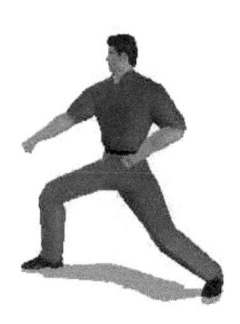

Straighten up as you bring the right arm across the body.

Step to the right with the right foot into a front stance as you execute a right low block.

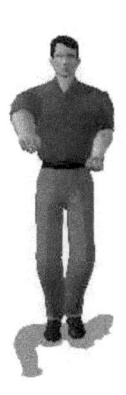

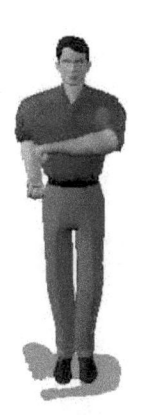

Bring the right foot back to the left foot. the right arm should swing as part of the whole body unit. The knees should be bent.

Straighten up as you bring the right arm back to the cocked position at the hip and swing the left arm across the body.

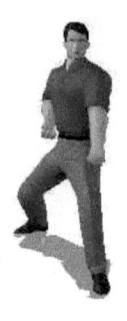

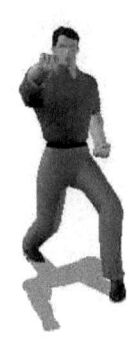

Step to the front with the left foot into a front stance as you execute a left low block.

Twist the right side of the body forward, the right foot pointing towards the left foot, as you execute a high right punch. you can drag the rear foot forward a little bit, but not too much. The whole body should be torqued a little bit.

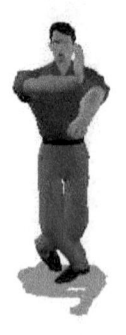

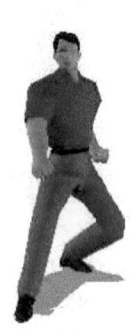

Step forward with the right foot to a x-stance. This is a precise movement where you ground with the right and bring the left foot up behind it at the same time. At the same time execute a left punch and a right cross palm.

Step back with the left foot into a back stance as you execute a right low block.

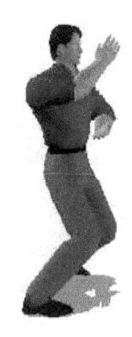

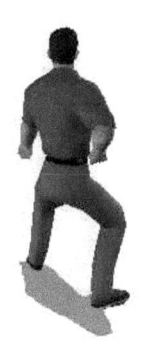

Pivot to the left into an hourglass stance as you protect the face with the right palm and prepare the left hand for a low block to the rear.

Continue pivoting to the left into a back stance as you execute a left low block.

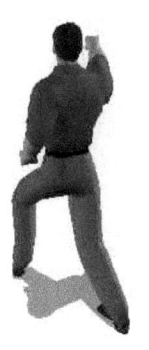

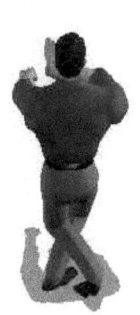

Twist to the left, drag the rear foot slightly, if you wish, but turn it towards the front foot. turning the foot will commit the hips, and therefore the whole weight, into the technique. At the same time as you twist, execute a right high punch.

Step forward with the right foot into an x-stance as you execute a left punch and a right cross palm block.

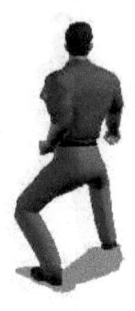

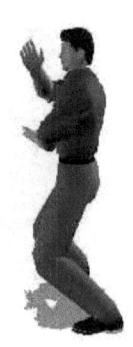

Step back with the left foot into a back stance as you execute a right low block.

Pivot to the left into a horse stance as you protect the face with the right hand and prepare the left hand.

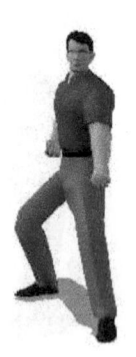

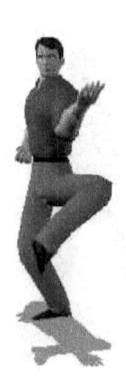

Continue pivoting to the left into a back stance as you execute a left low block.

Execute a left outward inverted knife hand block (open hand outward middle block) and a left sole block.

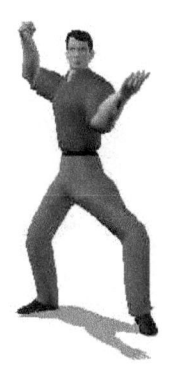

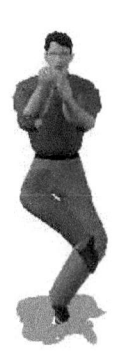

Step forward with the left foot as you raise the right fist in preparation for a right inward middle block.

Strike a right inward middle block against the open palm of the left hand as you execute a right sole block.

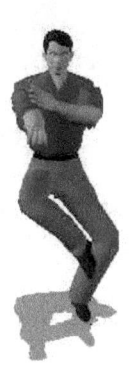

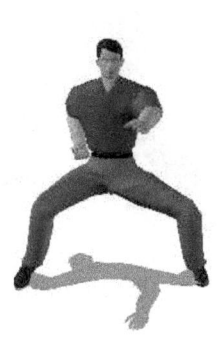

As you begin to move the right foot out (towards a horse) extend the right hand as you bring the left hand over the right arm.

Set into a horse stance with the right foot as you execute a left chop.

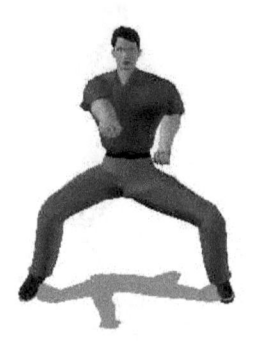

Execute a right punch.
Execute a left punch.

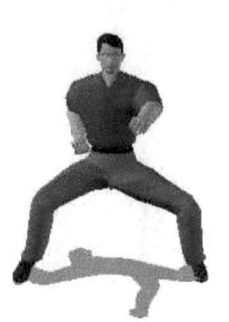

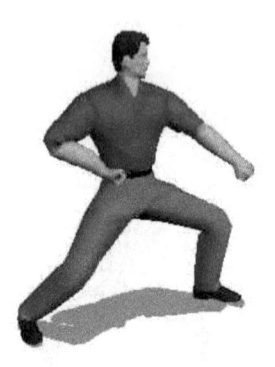

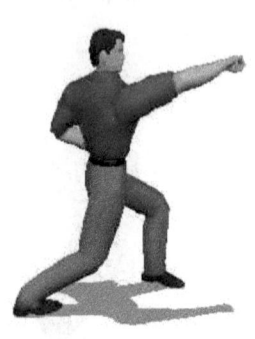

Stump the left leg back and to the left side into a front stance as you execute a left low block.

Twist to the left as you execute a left high punch.

Circle the hands down and around as you step forward with the right foot into a back stance and execute a right knife block.

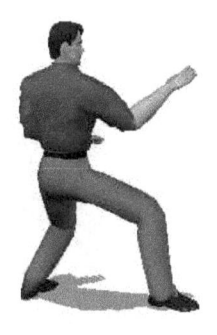

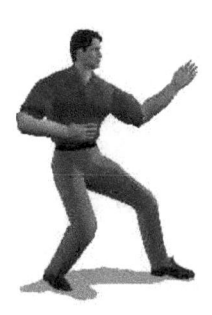

Drop the hands down and around as you step back with the right foot into a back stance and execute a left knife block.

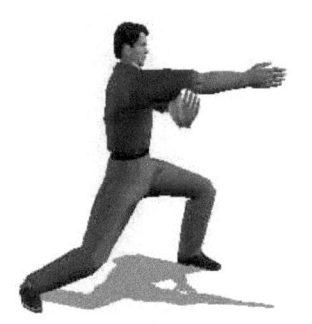

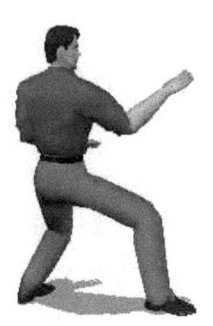

Shift forward into a front stance as you execute a right spear hand and a left cross palm block.

Circle the hands down and around as you step forward with the right foot into a back stance and execute a right knife block.

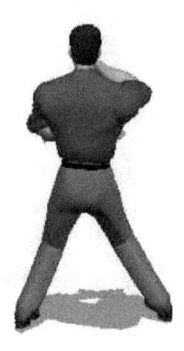

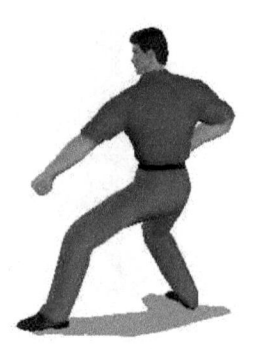

Pivot to the left into an hourglass stance as you protect the face with the right hand and prepare the left hand.

Continue the pivot to the left into a back stance as you execute a left low block.

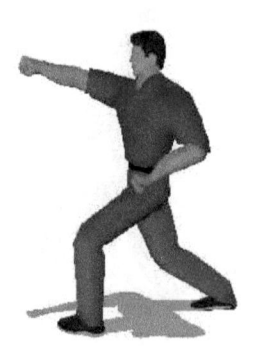

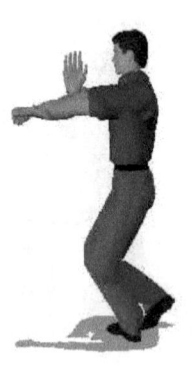

Twist to the left as you execute a high punch.

Step forward with the right foot into an x-stance as you execute a left punch and a right cross palm block.

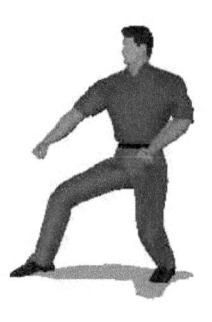

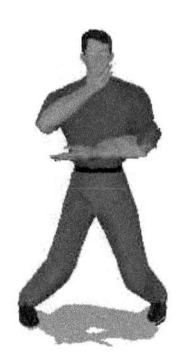

Step back with the left foot into a back stance as you execute a right low block.

Pivot to the left into a horse stance as you protect the face with the right hand and prepare the left hand.

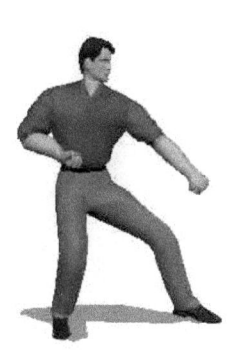

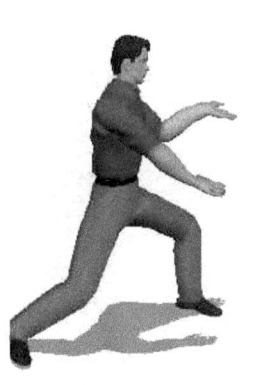

Continue the pivot to the left into a back stance as you execute a left low block.

Shift forward to a front stance as you execute a left upward palm block and a right downward palm block.

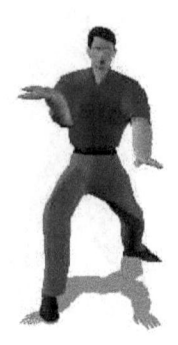

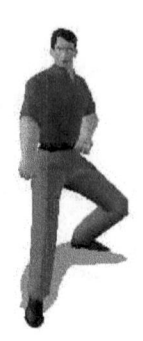

Step to the right with the right foot into a front stance as you execute a right upward palm block and a left downward palm block.

Shift back into a back stance as you execute a right low block.

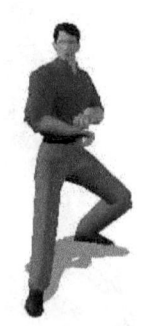

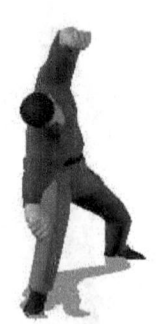

Bring the right hand back so that the back of the right fist is under the back of the left fist.

Shift forward into a front stance as you execute a right under punch and a left over punch.

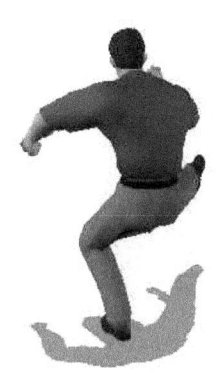

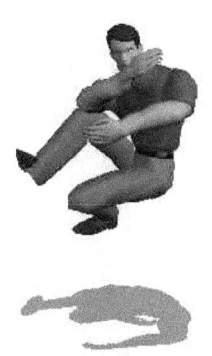

Pivot to the rear as you swing the right leg upwards and start to move the hands into a preparation position for a knife block.

Bring the left foot up as you spin in the air. The hands should be prepared for a knife block.

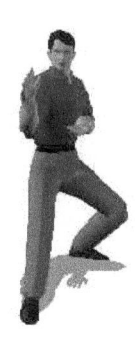

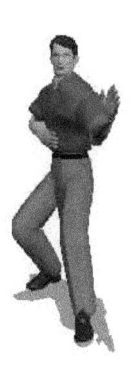

Land in a back stance with the right foot forward as you execute a right knife block.

Step back with the right foot into a back stance as you execute a left knife block.

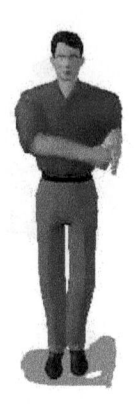

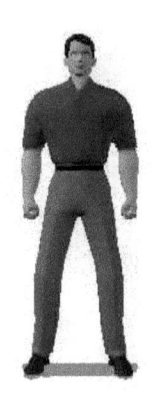

Step forward with the right foot until the feet are married. As you do so retract the knife hand and place the right fist against the left fingers. this is the beginning stance.

Step out with the right foot and assume a natural stance.

APPLICATION NUMBER FORTY-EIGHT

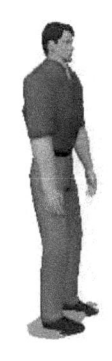

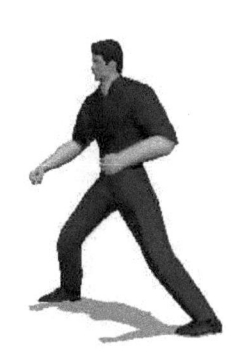

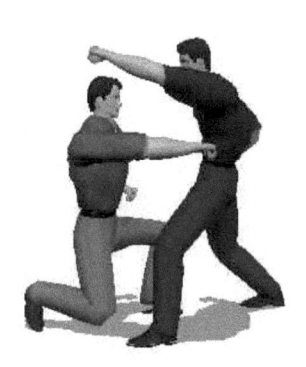

The Attacker prepares to punch.

The Attacker steps forward with the left foot into a front stance as he executes a left high punch. The Defender steps forward and slightly to the left into a kneeling stance as he executes a right punch.

The timing on this application is crucial. Move too soon and the Attacker will see what you are doing. Move too late and you're dead meat. This technique will aid you ability to see the thought behind your opponent's action, and to capitalize on it at exactly the right time.

Once you have accomplished CBM, and are using your body as one unit in everything you do, you will become aware that there is a higher level of CBM, which is called 2BCBM, which means Two Body Coordinated Body motion. 2BCBM requires that you CBM not only your own body, but that of your opponent.

APPLICATION NUMBER FORTY-NINE

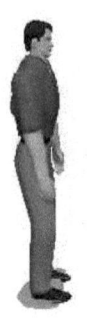

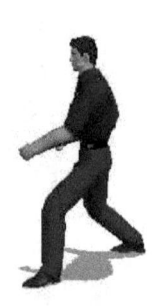

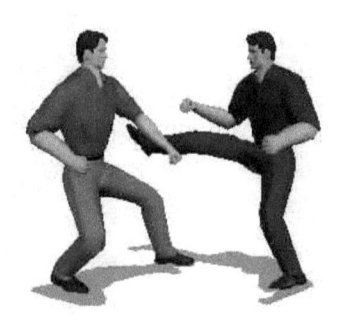

The Attacker prepares to kick.

The Attacker excutes a right kick. The Defender steps back with the right foot into a back stance as he executes a right low block.

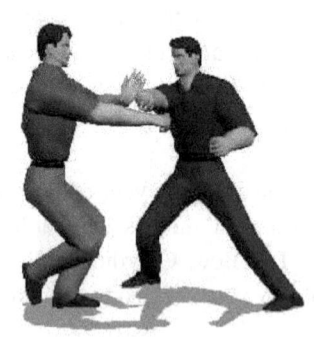

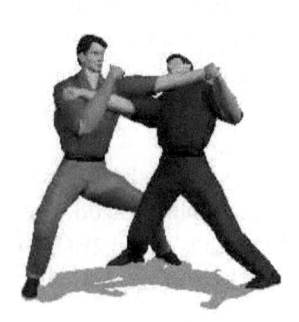

The Attacker sets his right foot forward in a front stance as he executes a right punch. The Defender brings the right foot behind the left foot as he executes a left cross palm block and a right punch.

The Defender steps forward (behind the Defender's right foot) with his left foot into a horse stance. the right arm traps the Attacker's right arm and the left hand arm goes across the Attacker's neck in a splitting technique. The Defender's left hand should be pointing, as this will increase intention and enhance the Coordinated Body Motion.

APPLICATION NUMBER FIFTY

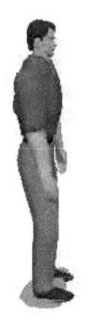

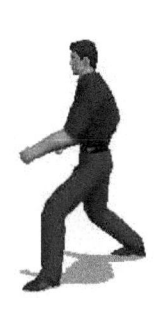

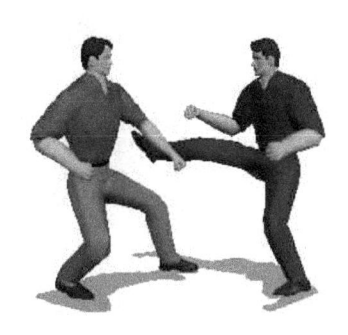

The Attacker prepares to kick.

The Attacker executes a right kick. The Defender steps back with the right foot into a back stance as he executes a right low block.

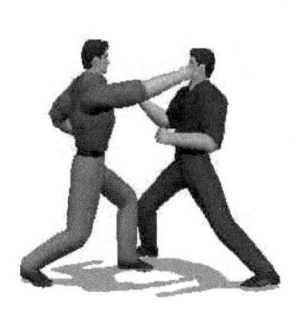

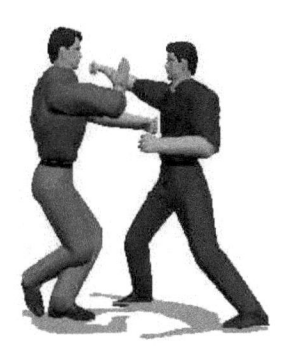

As the Attacker sets his right foot forward in a front stance the Defender shifts his weight forward and twists to the left as he executes a right punch to the face.

BUT, let's suppose the Attacker didn't set forward enough, or (horrors!) your punch didn't put him down. (More on this at the end of this application.) So the Attacker executes a right punch. The Defender moves the right foot behind the left foot in an x-stance as he executes a right cross palm and a left punch.

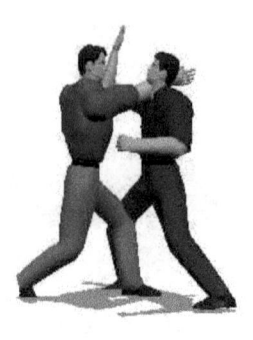

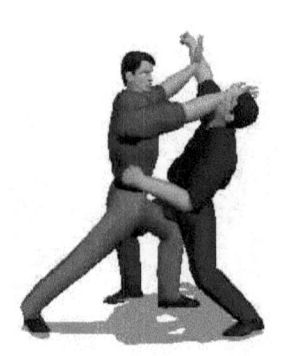

The Defender pushes the Attacker's right arm back with his left arm as he inserts the right arm against the side of the Attacker's neck.

The Defender pushes forward with stance as he begins pivoting to the right.

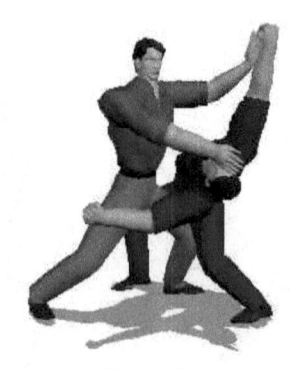

Yowza!

Okay, here's the skinny, Minny. The reason this application presents the concept that one punch might not put down an attacker is because, doggone it, it might not! The human body is a resilient thing. Attacker's do strange things, and, doggone it, no matter how dedicated you are to the concept of 'one punch-one kill,' it might not happen.

So don't give up the concept, practice harder, to make it work, but somewhere outside the thought of 'one punch-one kill' stared gently so it will not detract from your intention, is the idea that there must be a follow up technique.

THE IRON HORSE

This is also known as 'Tekki One,' or 'Kima Shodan,' and probably other names.

It is one of the most important forms in karate, as it gives to the student enormous amounts of power.

This form is supposed to be a practice for fighting from horseback, or side to side in rice paddies, and so on.

The real secret is that the stance is the most powerful one in karate.

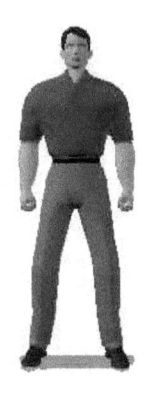

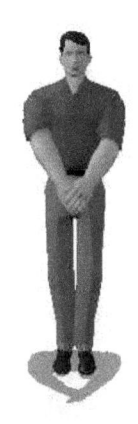

Assume a Natural Stance.

Bring the right foot in, place the left hand over the right in front of the groin.

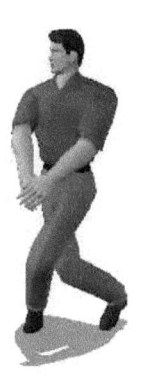

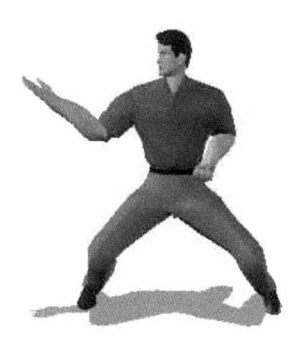

Step over the right foot to the right. The hips will turn a bit to the right. This is an x-stance, but is transitional.

Step to the side with right foot into a horse stance as you execute a right outward inverted knife hand block.

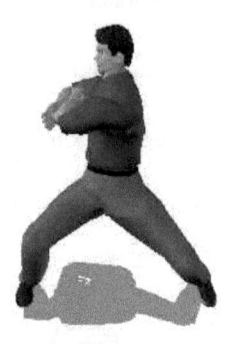

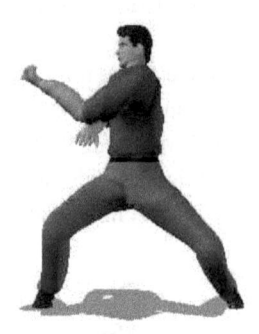

Execute a left elbow to the right palm to the right. Try not to twist the stance too much.

Lower the right hand slightly in a smothering palm as you execute a left backfist.

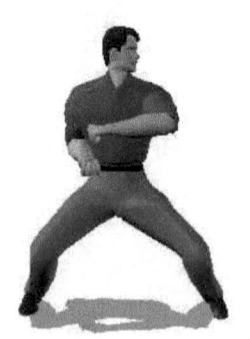

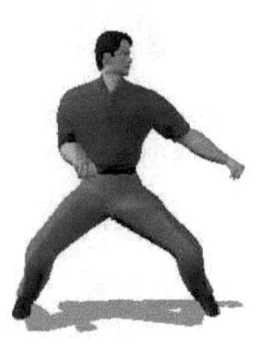

Turn the right palm over and make a fist in the cocked hip position. Simultaneously place the left fist (palm down over the right fist and turn the head to the left.

Execute a left low block to the left side.

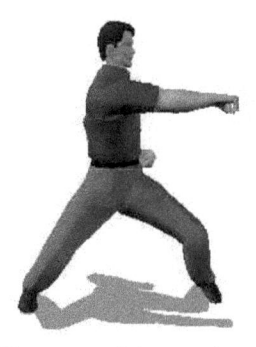

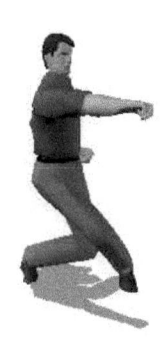

Execute a right punch to the left side.

Step to the left (over the right foot) with the left foot. This is a transitional x-stance. Your arm should start turning, joining with the hips in complete and utter CBM.

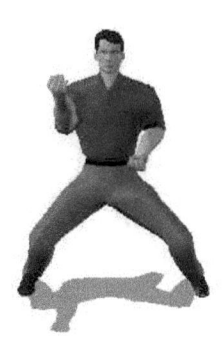

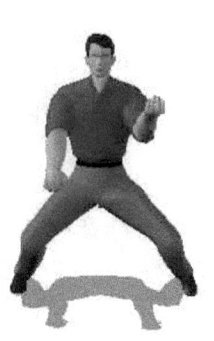

Step to the left (behind the left foot) with the right foot into a horse stance. The hips and middle outward block to the front should be simultaneous.

Execute a right low block and a left outward middle block.

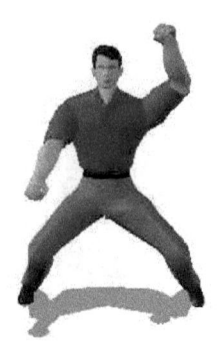

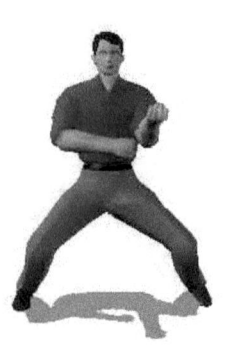

Raise the left hand to the left in a high block. Though this is a good block, the move should be done as if transitional.

Execute a left inward middle block. Bring the right fist to the augment position.

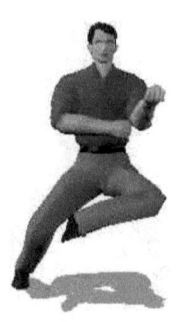

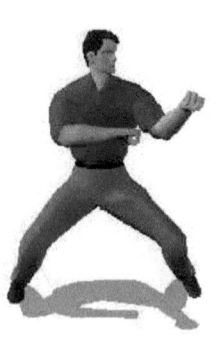

Execute a left sole block. This block must be done faster than you can fall.

Set down in the original horse stance position as you pivot the head to the left and execute a left inverted outward middle block.

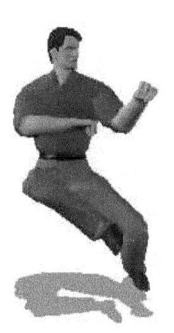

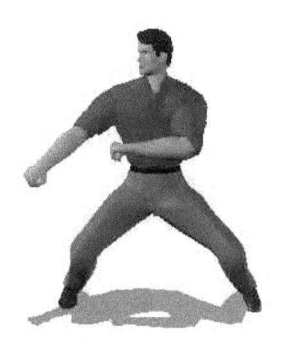

Execute a right sole block.
Set down in the original horse stance as you pivot the head to the right and execute a right low block.

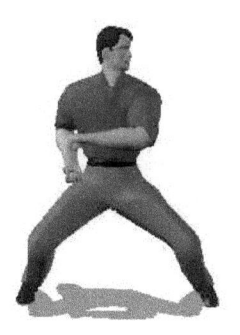

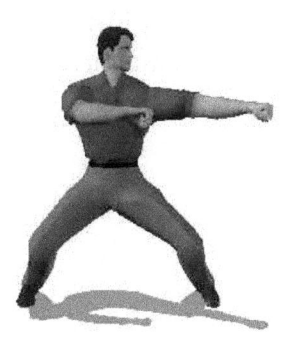

Prepare the hands on the right side of the body.
Execute punches to the left.

At this point you should execute an outward middle block to the left with the left hand. It will look exactly the opposite of the move illustrated in the fourth movement of this page. You are now going to do the form on the opposite side.

This is the way I prefer to teach it, as it makes the student manipulate the form in his mind.

Also, I don't teach applications for this form. It is the last form before black belt, so I ask the student to create three applications based on the movements of the form. Incidentally, as I mentioned in the beginning of this page, there are many variations on this form, yet the essence of it stays the same in most arts. That is because one can't argue with the basic power of the form.

About the Author

Al Case walked into his first martial arts school in 1967. During the Gold Age of Martial Arts he studied such arts as Aikido, Wing Chun, Ton Toi Northern Shaolin, Fut Ga Southern Shaolin, Weapons, Tai Chi Chuan, Pa Kua Chang, and others.

In 1981 he began writing for the martial arts magazines, including Inside Karate, Inside Kung Fu, Black Belt, Masters and Styles, and more.

In 1991 he was asked to write his own column in Inside Karate.

Beginning in 2001 he completed the basic studies of Matrixing, a logic approach to the Martial Arts he had been working on for over 30 years.

2011 he was heavily immersed in creating Neutronics, the science behind the science of Matrixing.

Interested martial artists can avail themselves of his research into Matrixing at MonsterMartialArts.com.

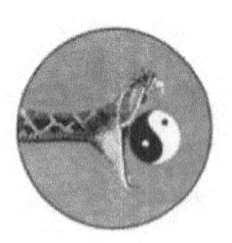

MonsterMartialArts.com

Did you know...

Al Case has written over forty novels?
Go to:

AlCaseBooks.com

Matrixing Kenpo Karate Series!

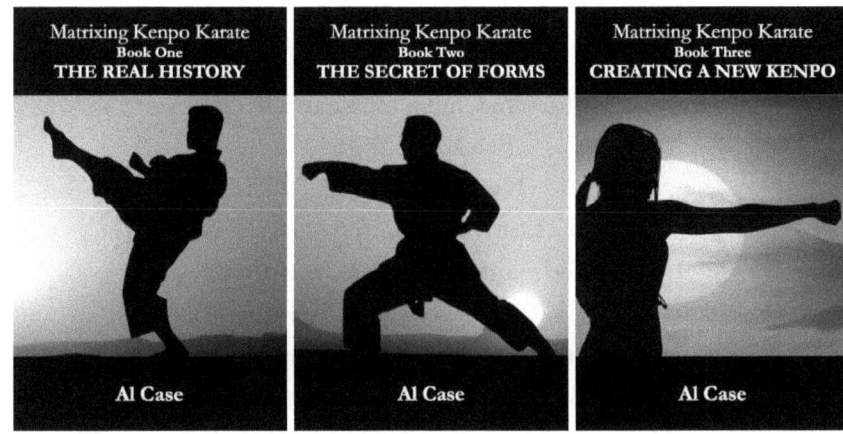

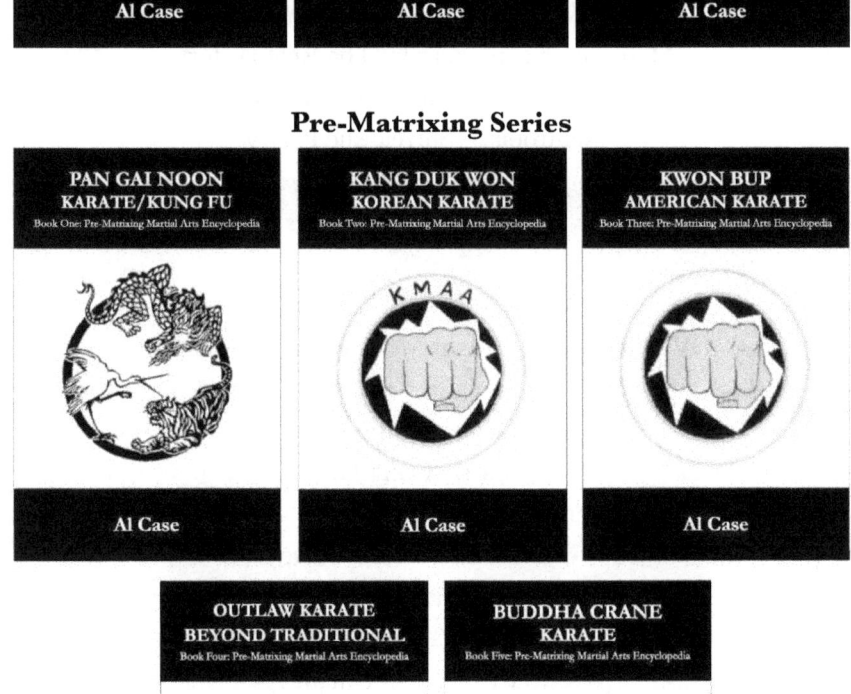

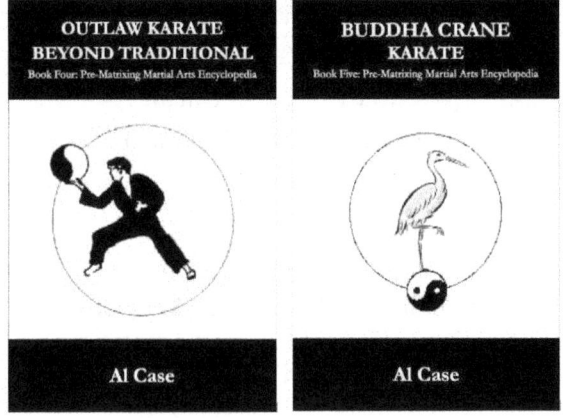

Matrixing Kenpo Karate, Book One: THE REAL HISTORY — Al Case

Matrixing Kenpo Karate, Book Two: THE SECRET OF FORMS — Al Case

Matrixing Kenpo Karate, Book Three: CREATING A NEW KENPO — Al Case

Pre-Matrixing Series

PAN GAI NOON KARATE/KUNG FU — Book One: Pre-Matrixing Martial Arts Encyclopedia — Al Case

KANG DUK WON KOREAN KARATE — Book Two: Pre-Matrixing Martial Arts Encyclopedia — Al Case

KWON BUP AMERICAN KARATE — Book Three: Pre-Matrixing Martial Arts Encyclopedia — Al Case

OUTLAW KARATE BEYOND TRADITIONAL — Book Four: Pre-Matrixing Martial Arts Encyclopedia — Al Case

BUDDHA CRANE KARATE — Book Five: Pre-Matrixing Martial Arts Encyclopedia — Al Case

MARTIAL ARTS BOOKS
On the internet

Advanced Tai Chi Chuan for Real Self Defense!
Black Belt Yoga
Five Martial Arts!
The Last Martial Arts Book (w video links!)
Hidden Techniques of Karate (w video links!)
How to Fix Karate (book one) (w video links!)
How to Fix Karate (book two) (w video links!)
Matrixing Kenpo Karate: Creating a New Kenpo
Matrixing Kenpo Karate: The Real History
Matrixing Kenpo Karate: The Secret of Forms
Neutropia ~ Surrealistic Poetry
The Book of Matrixing
The Book of Neutronics

VIDEO INSTRUCTION
DVDs and downloads at MonsterMartialArts.com

Matrix Karate
Matrix Kung Fu
Matrix Aikido
Master Instructor Course
Shaolin Butterfly
Butterfly Pa Kua Chang
Matrix Tai Chi Chuan
Five Army Tai Chi Chuan
Matrix Tai Chi Chuan
Five Army Tai Chi Chuan
Matrixing Kenjutsu
Blinding Steel (Matrixing Weapons)

Milton Keynes UK
Ingram Content Group UK Ltd.
UKHW022125051124
450708UK00015B/1188